THE PCOS WORKBOOK

YOUR GUIDE TO
COMPLETE PHYSICAL AND
EMOTIONAL HEALTH

THE

PCOS WORKBOOK

YOUR GUIDE TO COMPLETE PHYSICAL AND EMOTIONAL HEALTH

Angela Grassi, MS, RD, LDN
and Stephanie Mattei, Psy.D.

Luca Publishing
14 S. Bryn Mawr Avenue
Suite 204
Bryn Mawr, PA 19010
(484) 252-9028
www.PCOSnutrition.com

Leah Troiano, Editor

Cover design by Christine Davis

Text layout by Jonathan Gullery

The PCOS Workbook: Your Guide to Complete Physical and Emotional Health

Written by Angela Grassi and Stephanie Mattei

Manufactured in the United States of America

ISBN: 978-0-615-21784-0

CONTENTS

ACKNOWLEDGEMENTS

THIS workbook is a result of teamwork and we have many people on our team to thank. First, and most importantly, a special thank you to Leah Troiano for editing this book and making *The PCOS Workbook* the high quality book that it is. We are very proud of this workbook and know we couldn't have done it without her. Leah's skill, generosity, kindness and honesty are admirable. It was a pleasure to have you on our team. To Leah's husband Dave and her two beautiful daughters, Ella and Sophia: Thank you for sharing your wife and mother with us during this past year.

Dr. Mary Beth Ertel wrote the compassionate and comprehensive chapter, *Coping with Infertility*, which we know will help thousands of women who struggle with the challenges of infertility. *The PCOS Workbook* would not be complete without it. Thank you for agreeing to write this for us, especially as we both recognize the demands of being a new mother.

We'd also like to thank Christine Davis for designing yet another fantastic cover for our book. We admire your talent.

Angela Grassi: I would like to thank the many health professionals with whom I have the pleasure of collaborating. This includes Dr. Katherine Sherif and the staff at Drexel College of Medicine Center for PCOS; Dr. Stephen Somkuti and the physicians and staff at Abington Reproductive Medicine; Dr. Shahab Minassian; Dr. Jennifer Thie; and all the physicians at Main Line Fertility. Thank you for trusting me with your patients and thank you for the wonderful care you provide. You all inspire me to be the best dietitian I can be.

I also want to thank my husband Chris for his assistance, love and encouragement. I know I can do anything with him by my side. Thank you to Luca for putting up with his mom writing another book so soon after the first. I would also like to thank my family and friends for their endless support. I'm so lucky to have you all in my life.

This book would not exist without a collaboration with Dr. Stephanie Mattei. I want to thank Stephanie for all of her time, hard work, support, expertise and most of all her friendship. It has been such a pleasure to author *The PCOS Workbook* with her. She helped make the dream of a workbook for women with PCOS a reality.

Stephanie Mattei: Writing *The PCOS Workbook* has truly been an exciting experience. I have been honored to work with Angela in the past, and this project was just one more excuse to be in her company. Angela's love and passion for helping women with PCOS is inspiring. Her dedication to spreading knowledge and support is contagious. Without her excitement, this book could not have existed.

I also have to say that behind every great piece of work, is a great support system. Time, energy and attention spent on the book means time, energy and attention NOT spent somewhere else. For that I must thank my husband Angelo and my daughters Gabrielle and Samantha for giving me the space to make this project a priority. Your unconditional love, support and confidence is a gift.

Lastly, we'd like to thank all the women with PCOS with whom we've had the pleasure to work with. This book is for you.

Introduction

I wrote my first book, *The Dietitian's Guide to Polycystic Ovary Syndrome* to educate dietitians and other health care professionals about the importance of early recognition and treatment of PCOS. While I was writing it, I knew there should also be a book to help women manage this syndrome. As an expert in PCOS, I get numerous e-mails each day asking for advice, treatment, support and resources. The question was never, "Will I write a book for consumers?" but "When will it happen?" "What kind of book will it be?" and "Who else would author it?" I couldn't wait to get started.

Women with PCOS have different symptoms. Some of you have problems with weight, others struggle with infertility, and unfortunately, some of you struggle with both. I knew women with PCOS needed a book that could help them with all the different facets of PCOS. This included nutrition, stress management, mindful eating, infertility and body image. There are numerous books written about PCOS, yet none of them are written in a workbook form where you can explore and challenge specific difficulties you may experiencing. I am happy to say that I didn't have to wait long for my dream to become a reality. *The PCOS Workbook: Your Guide to Complete Physical and Emotional Health* naturally evolved through a collaborative process between Dr. Stephanie Mattei and me.

I met Dr. Mattei several years ago when we were part of a group treatment program for women with eating disorders. Dr. Mattei is a brilliant and passionate therapist who challenges her patients to live life without their eating disorders and to appreciate themselves for who they are. We instantly connected and worked well together.

Since her sister-in-law was diagnosed with PCOS, Dr. Mattei has been a passionate advocate for PCOS and learned everything she could about this complex and unique syndrome. Due to her strong background in treating mood disorders, food and body image issues plus her personal and professional experience with PCOS, I asked her to write the chapter "*Psychological Aspects of PCOS*" in my first book, *The Dietitian's Guide to Polycystic Ovary Syndrome*. From that point we started a monthly PCOS Psycho-Educational Support Group in the Philadelphia area. The group meetings provide a supportive, safe and informative setting for women to discuss and challenge their struggles. After gathering feedback from the groups, Dr. Mattei and I agreed that *The PCOS Workbook* was warranted. We wanted to give all women with PCOS the same support, education, resources and motivation to improve both your physical and emotional health. The ideas and exercises in *The PCOS Workbook* stem from group and individual sessions in response to the needs of our clients and others like you who struggle with PCOS. We hope you enjoy using this book as much as we've enjoyed creating it.

HOW TO USE THE PCOS WORKBOOK

The PCOS Workbook provides a place for you to explore your emotions and feelings about living with this syndrome and challenge the difficulties you face. We suggest you read this workbook from start to finish and complete each exercise. You will need a writing instrument and a highlighter (if you're the highlighting type) to complete the exercises (and for note taking). We encourage you to take your time with this workbook and not rush on to the next exercise or chapter. Remember: Making life changes is a process that evolves over time.

To manage PCOS, you must first understand it. Chapter 1, *Connecting the Dots: Understanding Polycystic Ovary Syndrome,* discusses what is really going on with your body when you have PCOS. This chapter discusses what insulin is and how it works as the catalyst to all the symptoms you experience. It also discusses the labs used to diagnose and monitor PCOS and treatment approaches.

Chapters 2 through 4 deal with the nutritional aspect of PCOS. In Chapter 2 you will learn about how food affects your insulin levels, which is key knowledge to make lasting changes in your health. Chapter 3, *Nutrition 411,* covers other nutritional concerns about PCOS, such as understanding food labels, portion sizes, nutritional supplements as well as effective grocery shopping and incorporating healthy foods into your diet. Chapter 4 asks you to analyze your food intake and exercise habits. Lastly, you will be asked to set and commit to nutrition goals to improve your health.

Chapter 5 is all about stress. It will walk you through identifying what "stressors" are in your life, explain how stress affects your body and offer techniques to proactively handle the stressors in your life.

Chapter 6, which tackles the topic of body image, will help you sort out the thoughts that interfere with living a more fulfilling life and then help you recognize the wonderful things your body has to offer.

In Chapter 7, we encourage you to try the concept of mindful eating. We identify emotional vs. mindless eating, and then teach you how to be mindful with food.

In Chapter 8, Dr. Mary Beth Ertel discusses *Coping with Infertility*. Dr. Ertel sheds light on the aloneness and frustration of infertility and provides an opportunity for you to process your feelings and emotions to better cope with this condition.

Lastly, the importance of managing PCOS to prevent the onset of other medical complications is discussed in Chapter 9.

We hope you enjoy *The PCOS Workbook* and that it helps you improve every aspect of your life.

Angela Grassi, MS, RD, LDN and *Dr. Stephanie Mattei, Psy.D*

This book is dedicated to
women with PCOS.

Chapter 1

Connecting the Dots: Understanding Polycystic Ovary Syndrome

DID you know that PCOS is one of the most complex endocrine disorders in the world? Understanding what's going on with your body and why will help you to properly manage PCOS, both physically and emotionally.

This chapter discusses:

- What PCOS is and the connection with insulin resistance,
- The criteria physicians use to diagnose PCOS,
- Labs used to diagnose and monitor PCOS, and
- Treatment approaches.

Before you read this chapter, take time to write down questions you have about your diagnosis and your health. These could be general questions about medical terms you've heard, lab tests you need or more detailed questions about what's going on with your body. Then, as you obtain your answers from this workbook, revisit your questions and answer them in the space provided. If you still need clarification, take your questions to your health care professional.

Questions I have about PCOS:

1. _Why am I so scatter brained ?_____ ?

Answer:

_____

_____

_____

2. <u>Why do I feel so anxious?</u> ?

Answer:

_____

_____

_____

3. <u>Depression - 3years into Diagnosis - Awful</u>

Answer:

_____

_____

_____

4. _____ ?

Answer:

_____

_____

_____

5. _____ ?

Answer:

_____

_____

_____

WHAT EXACTLY IS PCOS?

PCOS is both an endocrine and reproductive disorder that affects one out of every 10 women in the United States. Recognized in 1935 by scientists Irving F. Stein and Michael Leventhal for its relationship to menstrual disturbances, PCOS was primarily viewed as a reproductive disorder. However, due to its insulin resistance component, PCOS is now viewed mainly as an endocrine disorder. PCOS is characterized by high levels of androgens or male sex hormones and problems with ovulation. But, to fully understand PCOS, you must first learn about the role key hormones play in the syndrome.

Insulin: The key to it all

Insulin is a growth hormone that we all need to survive. Insulin transports glucose (our body's main source of fuel) from our bloodstream into our cells where it can be used as energy. For example, when you eat a granola bar your body breaks it down into small glucose particles that enter your bloodstream. In response, insulin is secreted and used to carry the glucose into your cells to be used for energy (see Figure 1.0).

Sometimes insulin's role in your body is explained by using a lock and key analogy. There are locked doors on our cell walls and insulin is the key. The only way glucose can enter cells is by opening the locks. Insulin acts as a key to open the door to the cells to allow glucose to enter.

The spare tire

If you have been diagnosed with PCOS, chances are you have insulin resistance. This occurs when your cell doors do not respond appropriately to the normal amounts of insulin produced by your body. In other words, your insulin "key" does not fit well into the "lock" on your cells walls. When this happens, extra insulin is produced to increase the chances of getting more glucose into your cells (see Figure 1.0). The result: Your body has too much insulin.

Figure 1.0. The difference between a normal cell and insulin resistant cell.

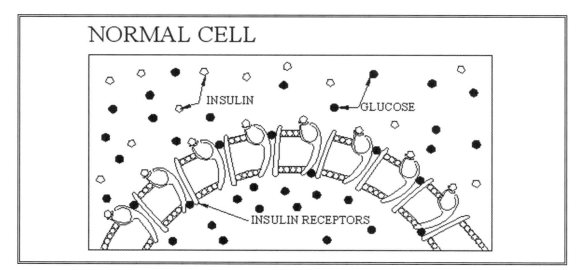

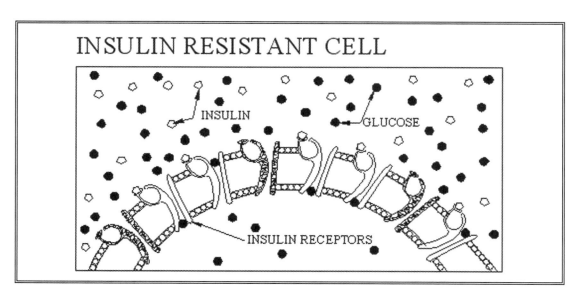

Since insulin is a growth hormone, too much promotes weight gain, mostly in your midsection, above your belly button resembling a "spare tire." If you are gaining lots of weight without significant changes to diet or exercise, excess insulin could be the culprit. The weight is gained despite appropriate physical activity and caloric intake. Because women who are overweight are likely to experience more insulin resistance than those who are not, elevated insulin and weight gain create a vicious cycle. The more weight you gain, the more corresponding insulin your body produces, and the more you gain weight (see Figure 1.1).

Figure 1.1. The vicious cycle of insulin resistance.

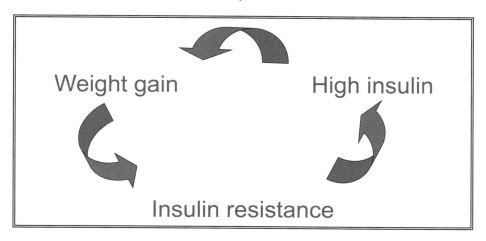

Besides weight gain, insulin resistance can cause many other changes:

- Skin tags,
- Follicular keratosis or reddened, rough hair follicles on the upper arms,
- Dry and rough elbows, or dirty looking patches of skin called acanthosis nigricans, a Latin term for "dark skin." The patches are usually found behind the neck; on the elbows, knees, underarms; between the breasts and across the knuckles and groin. In people with lighter skin, acanthosis nigricans may manifest as tan-colored skin above the neckline and rough gray elbows. The greater the amount of insulin, the more severe the acanthosis nigricans.

Other symptoms of insulin resistance include hypoglycemia (or low blood sugar) and strong, almost urgent, cravings for carbohydrates and sweets. Hypoglycemia can occur if you wait too long to eat. It can also happen if you have a meal or snack containing mostly refined carbohydrates (like pasta or candy) and too little protein. When a large amount of glucose enters your bloodstream at once, the body responds by releasing a large amount of insulin. Insulin quickly puts the glucose into your cells, leaving your blood low in glucose. The following symptoms are sometimes experienced: hunger, fatigue, nausea, shakiness, irritability, dizziness or headaches.

A fast insulin release followed by low blood sugar may also explain why many women have a strong desire for sweets and intense cravings. When your blood sugar drops, your blood glucose is low and your brain tells your body it needs more glucose now! To raise blood sugar levels, your body tells you to eat. After eating, glucose enters your blood stream quickly giving you a rapid rise in blood sugar, which makes you feel better. The more refined food you eat, the greater increase in insulin and the more refined foods you crave. Simply, the more sugar you eat, the more you want. To avoid low blood sugar, eat small, balanced meals often. Limit refined food and include sufficient protein in each meal or snack to slow the release of sugar. You'll learn more about balancing food choices in the next two chapters.

If not well managed, over time, elevated insulin levels may lead to type 2 diabetes as the insulin receptors on the cell walls become more resistant, eventually ignoring the insulin. This result: Excess glucose stays in the bloodstream affecting blood circulation and causing long-term tissue damage.

All about androgens

Androgens are male sex hormones such as testosterone and dehydroepiandrosterone sulfate (DHEA-sulfate). Women also have androgens, just like men have female hormones like estrogen. Unlike men, when insulin levels become elevated in women with PCOS, the ovaries are stimulated to produce more androgens. This affects the balance of female sex hormones that control your menstrual cycle, most notably increasing luteinizing hormone (LH) and decreasing follicle-stimulating hormone (FSH). The imbalance may affect ovulation. Eggs that are meant to be released and fertilized for conception aren't able to mature and release and instead become small, fluid-filled sacks or cysts that surround your ovaries (hence the term, poly "cystic" ovary). The cysts are a result of hormonal imbalances, not the cause of them. The imbalance of sex hormones can result in you having absent menstrual periods for months at a time or irregular ones (menstrual cycles longer than 42 days or several periods in one month). Some women with PCOS will have monthly cycles, but, may bleed heavily. Figure 1.2 summarizes the affect of high insulin on androgens and menstrual cycle.

Figure 1.2. The affect elevated insulin has on androgens and menstrual cycle.

Insulin resistance → high insulin →↑↑ androgens → irregular, heavy, absent menstrual cycles

An overproduction of androgens in women can result in the following: Excessive hair growth on the face and body (hirsutism), balding (alopecia), acne and other skin problems, all of which can have a negative impact on your body image and self-esteem, and are covered more in Chapter 6.

A lot of information has been presented so far! At this point, take time to process what you have just read. Write down key points or summarize what you have learned.

_____

_____

_____

_____

_____

_____

_____

_____

_____

_____

_____

_____

What causes PCOS?

The actual cause of PCOS is unknown. However, current research is directed at finding out why it occurs. Genetics play a part, as many women with PCOS have female relatives on either the maternal or paternal side with a history of irregular periods and/or infertility. Researchers have found polycystic-appearing ovaries in young girls before and after puberty. Some research indicates the possibility that baby girls are born with polycystic ovaries. Still, more theories suggest that women may develop PCOS from being exposed to high androgen (testosterone) levels in the womb.

How is PCOS diagnosed?

A formal diagnostic criteria for PCOS is lacking. Instead, physicians use an agreed upon criteria to diagnose PCOS. A woman can be diagnosed with PCOS if she has two of the following three criteria (with the exclusion of any other medical problems):

- Irregular periods or no periods (less than eight menstrual cycles per year),

- Blood tests or physical signs of high androgens (elevated testosterone, excessive hair growth, balding, acne),
- The presence of cysts surrounding the ovary (upon an ultrasound).

If you are taking birth control medications to regulate your menstrual cycle, they may lower androgens, making PCOS difficult to diagnose. Be sure to let your doctor know if you are taking any birth control medications. In addition, a small percentage of women with PCOS have monthly periods, but experience very heavy bleeding and sometimes pass clots. One other problem with these criteria is that about 25% of women with PCOS don't get cysts. Even with the criteria, diagnosing PCOS may still be difficult.

KNOW YOUR NUMBERS

Lab tests help your physician diagnose and monitor your PCOS. They can also indicate how well your body is functioning or signal something wrong with your health, so it's important that you keep them for your records and for comparison later on. Ask your doctor's office for a copy or request that the lab send you the results directly. Your results record the blood work your physician ordered. You can also use your lab reports to compare levels with previous results, tracking improvements or worsening conditions such as your cholesterol or blood sugar levels. Be aware that optimal ranges are provided in your lab reports along with your results. They can differ slightly depending on the lab that processes your blood work so try to use the same lab each time you get your blood drawn. A record-keeping form for your lab results is provided in the appendix. The following are a sampling of lab tests that physicians may use to help diagnose and monitor PCOS:

1. **Total testosterone** measures the total amount of testosterone your body produces including free and bound testosterone levels. Elevated levels are ≥ 50 ng/dl.
2. **Luteinizing hormone (LH)** measures the amount of LH in your body. LH plays a role in egg development and release. Usually, LH levels are elevated in women with PCOS.
3. **Follicle stimulating hormone (FSH)** measures FSH in your body. FSH is responsible for egg maturation. Levels can be normal or low in women with PCOS.
4. **LH:FSH ratio** compares levels of LH to FSH. Many (but not all) women with PCOS have abnormal FSH to LH ratios. Normally this ratio is about 1:1, meaning the FSH and LH levels in the blood are similar. In women with PCOS, the LH to FSH ratio is often higher, for example 2:1 or even 3:1.
5. **DHEA-sulfate** is an androgen. This test detects how much androgens or male hormones your body is producing. DHEA-sulfate gets converted into testosterone. This test also rules out adrenal problems, which can mimic PCOS symptoms.
6. **Prolactin** is a hormone secreted from the pituitary gland. This test is used to rule out a prolactin-secreting pituitary tumor.
7. **Thyroid-stimulating hormone (TSH)** is a blood test used to assess thyroid functioning. A hypothyroid indicates a slow metabolism and causes elevated TSH levels, possibly

indicating thyroid damage. A hyperthyroid may indicate a faster metabolism resulting in low levels of TSH in the blood. Normal levels of TSH are .4 to 2.5 IU/mL.

8. **Liver function tests (LFTs)** are used to monitor liver function. They include the liver enzymes AST and ALT. Since all medications pass through the liver, monitoring the liver function every three to six months is essential. Elevated LFT levels indicate liver damage.

9. **Fasting lipid profile includes:**

   - **Total Cholesterol** or the total amount of cholesterol in your body. Ideal is < 200 mg/dL.
   - **High-density lipoproteins (HDL)** or the good cholesterol. The higher the better. Ideal is > 55 mg/dL. You are at a higher risk for heart disease with low levels of HDL.
   - **Low-density lipoproteins (LDL)** or the bad cholesterol. Optimal is < 100 mg/dL. The higher your level of LDL, the greater your risk for heart disease and stroke.
   - **Triglycerides (TG)** or fat in your bloodstream. Ideal level is < 150 mg/dL.

   Note: having lipid levels outside of normal ranges puts you at a higher risk for heart disease.

10. **Fasting insulin** is used to detect elevated insulin levels or insulin resistance. A fasting insulin blood test may be performed alone or as part of an oral glucose tolerance test (a test that measures your fasting glucose at various intervals after consuming a sugary drink). When tested every three to six months, fasting insulin can assess the use of insulin-lowering medications or dietary changes. Fasting insulin tests require a frozen specimen, meaning the blood is frozen immediately after it's drawn and remains frozen until tested. Erroneously low levels may result if your blood is not kept frozen. Your physician's office may not be equipped to freeze blood and you may need to take this test in a different location. Your fasting insulin should be < 10 IU/mL.

11. **Fasting blood glucose** measures the amount of glucose (sugar) in your blood. Ideally, levels should be between 70-99 mg/dL. Diabetes is diagnosed when fasting glucose levels are > 126 mg/dL.

12. **Fasting glucose to insulin ratio** is used to diagnose and monitor insulin resistance by determining the level of fasting glucose compared to the level of fasting insulin. A glucose to insulin ratio of less than 4:5 usually indicates insulin resistance.

13. **Hemoglobin A1C (HA1C)** measures long-term blood sugar levels during a three-month period. Optimal levels should be < 6%.

14. **Vitamin D** measures the amount of vitamin D in blood. Optimal levels should be > 35 ng/dL.

15. **High-sensitivity C-reactive protein (hsCRP)** measures your level of C-reactive protein, which is a marker of inflammation. Levels ≥ 3 mg/L increase your cardiac risk.

PCOS LAB RESULTS TRACKING FORM

Lab Test	Optimal Levels	Date: Result	Date: Result	Date: Result	Date: Result	Date: Result	Date: Result	Date: Result	Date: Result
Total Cholesterol	< 200 mg/dL								
LDL	< 100 mg/dL								
HDL	> 55 mg/dL								
Triglycerides	< 150 mg/dL								
Fasting Glucose	70-99 mg/dL								
HA1C	< 6%								
Fasting Insulin	< 10 IU/mL								
Fasting Glucose:Insulin	> 4:5								
Total Testosterone	< 50 ng/dL								
LH	_____								
FSH	_____								
LH:FSH	1:1								
Vitamin D	> 35 ng/dL								
TSH	.4-2.5 IU/mL								
hsCRP	< 3 mg/L								
Blood Pressure	< 120/80 mmHg								

GOALS OF TREATMENT

Treatment should address both the reproductive and metabolic disturbances of PCOS and include maintaining or reducing your weight, decreasing insulin and androgens, preventing or treating cardiovascular risk factors and improving your reproductive function. Improving insulin resistance will have favorable affects on both fertility and metabolic aspects, and can assist in weight loss. Treatment options for insulin resistance are diet, physical activity and insulin-lowering medications (see below).

MEDICATIONS

Since not all women with PCOS experience the same symptoms or severity of symptoms, treatment approaches can differ. The following are the most common types of medications used to improve various aspects of PCOS. Office visits will vary depending upon your physician but most likely occur every three to six months to evaluate the effectiveness of the medications, especially in the beginning of treatment.

Oral contraceptives. These are birth control medications taken in pill form. Benefits include regular menstruation, improvement in acne, balding and hair growth due to better hormone regulation. Risk factors of oral contraceptives include blood clots, increased triglycerides and insulin resistance (in some brands).

Anti-androgens. These medications work to decrease the amount of androgens (male sex hormones). The most common medications are Flutamide® (Eulexin™) and Spironolactone® (Aldactone™). Anti-androgens work by competing for absorption with testosterone receptors. They usually require three to six months to take effect but results can be dramatic in improving hair growth, acne and balding.

Spironolactone has been found to cause birth defects and should not be used by women trying to conceive. Side effects of Spironolactone include nausea, diarrhea, headaches, dizziness and menstrual cycle irregularities (frequent monthly bleeding or no bleeding). Side effects of Flutamide can include nausea, diarrhea, hot flashes and reduced fertility.

INSULIN-LOWERING MEDICATIONS

Metformin® (Glucophage®, Bristol-Myers Squibb Co.) (also called Glumetza® or Fortamet®) is an insulin-lowering medication. The most common medication used to treat PCOS, Metformin is effective at improving cholesterol and blood pressure, lowering blood glucose, insulin and testosterone and is helpful with weight management. This drug also increases ovulation so if you don't want to conceive, you must use contraception.

Side effects include abdominal bloating, gas, nausea and diarrhea. Usually, if you start with a lower dose or take Metformin with food, the side effects may be minimal. For most women, side effects subside after the first several weeks of use. Some women may prefer the extended released version (XR or ER), which tends to have the least amount of side effects. Eating refined carbohydrates may cause an increase in diarrhea and nausea. Within a few days of starting Metformin, some women report a decrease in carbohydrate cravings and less hypoglycemia.

Metformin lowers blood glucose levels in three ways: (1) it suppresses the liver's production of glucose, (2) increases your body's sensitivity to insulin and (3) decreases the absorption of carbohydrates. Metformin is now being offered to women with PCOS during pregnancy to prevent gestational diabetes and possibly decrease the risk of miscarriage. Taking Metformin requires maintaining a balanced diet and regular physical activity to see effects.

Thiazolidenediones (TZDs). This group of medications is a class of insulin-lowering drugs, such as Actos® (Pioglitazone, Takeda Pharmaceuticals North America, Inc.) that can be used alone or in conjunction with Metformin to improve insulin levels and cardiovascular risk, reduce androgen levels and hirsutism. TZDs work to increase the efficiency of insulin receptors. If taking Metformin, and making changes to your diet and exercise patterns do not garner results, adding of TZDs may be more effective. TZDs may cause some initial water retention.

Byetta®. This medication helps people with diabetes control blood glucose levels. Although still not indicated for PCOS, some physicians use Byetta alone or in conjunction with Metformin or TZDs to help PCOS patients manage insulin levels and possibly lose weight. Byetta is injected via a pen in pre-measured dosage. It helps your body produce the proper amount of insulin after you eat, stops the liver from producing too much glucose when your body doesn't need it and slows the rate that food leaves your stomach, which prevents spikes in insulin. Byetta is taken before meals. Common side effects are nausea and decreased interest in food.

Use the space provided to write notes or questions to discuss with your doctor:

_____

_____

_____

_____

_____

_____

_____

DIET AND EXERCISE

Finally, in addition to medication, you must change your eating and lifestyle to improve your health, fertility and weight. Improvements in your eating patterns can reduce your insulin and androgen levels, and increase your ovulation. This includes eating a balanced diet for PCOS along with regular physical activity. The next three chapters offer information and support to take control of your eating and your physical health.

CHAPTER 2

HOW FOOD AFFECTS YOUR INSULIN LEVELS

DID you know the majority of food we eat is made up of carbohydrates? Fruit, vegetables, whole grains, legumes (beans, lentils and peas) and milk all contain carbohydrates. While they play different roles in a healthy PCOS diet, not all carbohydrates are considered equal. Although foods containing fat and protein affect insulin levels, carbohydrates have the most impact. Since your body produces too much insulin, the focus of treatment for PCOS is lowering those insulin levels. Therefore, your main mission is choosing foods that don't contribute to raising (especially rapidly) your insulin levels.

In this section, we will discuss different types of carbohydrates, their benefits, how they affect insulin levels and how they fit into a healthy meal plan. The PCOS Food Exchange List found on page 36 outlines what foods contain carbohydrates and proper portion size. A copy of the PCOS Food Exchange List is located in the appendix.

THE BALANCING ACT

Figure 2.0 shows how different foods affect your insulin levels. Simple and refined carbohydrates cause rapid rises in insulin whereas the other "slow" carbohydrate-containing foods (whole grains, fruits, vegetables and milk) gradually increase insulin keeping blood sugar levels more stable. While "slow" is the way to go, exercise caution when eating them as eating too much at once will raise your insulin levels. The entire left side of the PCOS Food Exchange List indicates foods that contain carbohydrates (grains and starches, fruits, starchy vegetables and non-starchy vegetables), amount of carbohydrates in grams and appropriate portion sizes. A slice of whole wheat bread has the same amount of carbohydrates as a small apple (15 grams). Thus, you will need to balance the amount and type of carbohydrates you have with your meals and snacks. To avoid surges in insulin levels, limit your carbohydrate intake to one to three servings per meal (15-45 grams of total carbohydrates) and one to two per snack (15-30 grams of total carbohydrates). Although still important, protein and fat do not contain carbohydrates and affect insulin levels to a lesser extent. They are discussed later in this chapter. Meal plans using these guidelines are located in the appendix.

Figure 2.0. **The affect of food on insulin levels.**

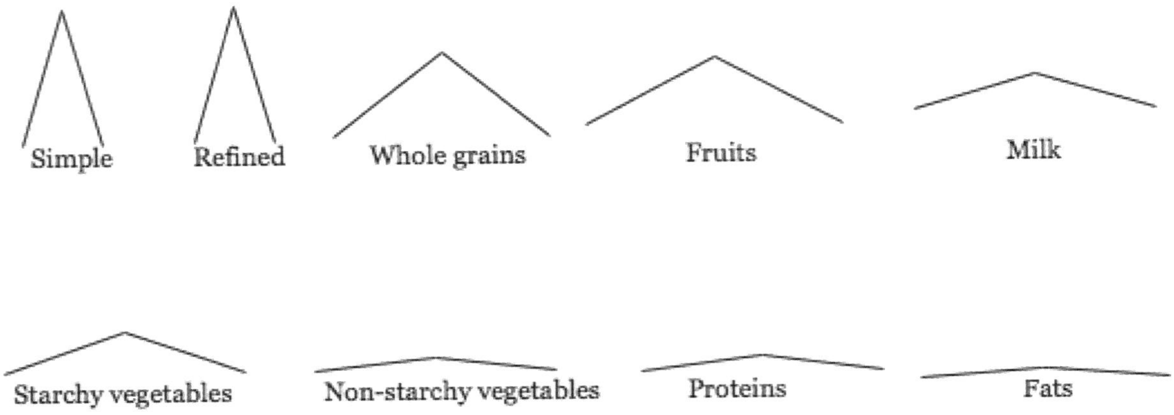

Figure 2.0 shows how different foods affect insulin levels. Simple and refined carbohydrates cause rapid rises in insulin whereas whole grains, fruits, vegetables and milk gradually increase insulin levels. Protein and fat affect insulin to a lesser extent.

AVOID THE INSULIN SURGE

Simple carbohydrates are carbohydrates broken down into very refined or tiny glucose particles. This means the body doesn't have to work hard to break them down. Because of this, they enter the bloodstream immediately causing a rapid rise in blood sugar, which triggers a rapid increase in insulin. Notice in Figure 2.0 how steep the spike of simple carbohydrates is compared to other carbohydrate containing foods.

Eating simple carbohydrates worsens PCOS by raising insulin levels and contributing to weight gain. Examples of simple carbohydrate foods include candy, baked goods, sweetened beverages (i.e., soda, iced tea, juice), honey and sugar. Simple carbohydrates wreak havoc in a PCOS body, so do your best to eliminate simple carbohydrates from your diet.

Refined carbohydrates are similar to simple carbohydrates, but they require more processing during digestion to be used as glucose. Refined carbohydrates started out as whole grains but were refined during the manufacturing process by removing the outer layers of the whole grain. This process extends the shelf life of food and alters its taste and texture. The outer layers of the grain contain most of the vitamins and minerals. When these outer layers are stripped, manufacturers will typically "enrich" the product by adding back some of the lost nutrients. Fiber is also found in the outer layers but unlike the nutrients, fiber is not replaced. Therefore, refined carbs are not the best food choice for women with PCOS.

To find the best choice for your body, which is whole grains, you must read food labels. If the word "whole" is missing from the first ingredient in the ingredient list (such as wheat flour instead of whole wheat flour), the food is refined. Examples of refined foods include white bread, white pasta, white rice, low-fiber cereal (i.e. Cornflakes™, Rice Krispies™, Special K™, Fruit Loops™) and various granola bars. The first ingredient in these products reads "enriched wheat flour." Because refined carbohydrates don't contain fiber or the nutrient profile of a whole grain, they offer little nutritional value. Like simple carbohydrates, refined foods raise insulin levels as they enter the bloodstream rapidly causing a surge in insulin and worsening insulin resistance (see Figure 2.0). Women with PCOS don't need to completely eliminate refined foods from their diet, but should eat them in limited quantities such as once or twice a week.

Can you name some of your favorite foods that fall into the simple or refined carbohydrate category?

Simple   **Refined**

_____   _____

_____   _____

_____   _____

_____   _____

_____   _____

Slow carbs rule!

Unrefined or whole-grain carbohydrates. A whole grain consists of three layers: The bran, the endosperm and the germ (see Figure 2.1). Often the outer two layers, the bran and the endosperm, are removed to produce a refined product. Phytochemicals, antioxidants and fiber present in the whole grain are not added back to the refined grain. If the grain doesn't go through the refining process and its three layers remain intact, it's considered a "whole grain."

Figure 2.1. The three layers of a whole grain.

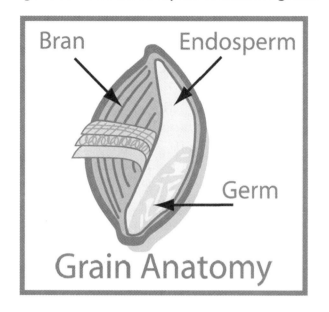

Courtesy of Bob's Red Mill and the Whole Grains Council

All grains begin as whole grains. Wheat, corn, oats, rye and barley are common whole grains consumed in the United States. Other grains such as spelt, millet, kamut and quinoa are rapidly rising in popularity among health-conscious consumers. In fact, most if not all of these grains can be found on the shelves of any grocery store. (Whole Foods™ has some grains located in large bins in the front of its store, making them hard to miss.)

Research has shown that eating whole grains improves insulin resistance, supporting the need for them in the PCOS diet. Whole grains can improve insulin resistance by slowing the release of glucose and preventing large insulin spikes (see Figure 2.0). Insulin levels also improve by consuming nutrients found in whole grains, such as chromium, magnesium and selenium. These nutrients along with dietary fiber, phytochemicals and antioxidants found in whole grains can also decrease the risk of cancer and diabetes.

Whole grains are heart healthy, too. Not only do whole grains lower cholesterol and trig-lyceride levels, there's also a strong correlation between the consumption of whole grains and a decreased risk of developing heart disease and high blood pressure.

Daily consumption of whole grains may also help with weight management as whole grains slow the digestion and absorption of carbohydrates and give a sense of fullness that lasts longer than refined grains.

Write down whole grains that you enjoy eating:

_____   _____

_____   _____

_____   _____

_____   _____

_____   _____

HOW MANY GRAINS SHOULD I EAT?

The U.S. Dietary Guidelines suggest that whole grains make up at least half of your grain intake. However, women with PCOS should choose whole grains 100% of the time. The PCOS Food Exchange List shows portion sizes of whole grains. The following are some examples of these serving sizes (1 ounce each):

- 1/2 cup cooked cereal, pasta or rice = a small computer mouse
- 1 cup dry cereal = a baseball
- 1 tortilla= a small (6 inch) salad plate
- 1 pancake or waffle = a music CD

Just because whole grains are healthy doesn't mean you can eat as many as you want. Large amounts will spike your insulin levels. To avoid spiking, eat whole grains spread out evenly throughout the day, perhaps one to three servings at each meal or snack instead of eating a day's worth of grains at once. You should consume whole grains that are low in sugar and combine protein with these grains to slow the release of insulin as protein slows the release of glucose. For example, a meal can consist of 4 to 6 ounces of grilled fish, 2/3 cup cooked brown rice, non-starchy vegetables and a salad with low-sugar dressing. Sample menus are provided in the appendix. If you are interested in learning more about your body's specific carbohydrate needs, consult a registered dietitian.

PCOS FOOD EXCHANGE LIST

Items on the left side of page, consume between 1–3 servings per meal and 1-2 servings per snack.*

GRAINS & STARCHES:
(15 grams carbohydrate each)
Whole grain, high fiber, low sugar are best.
1 slice of whole grain bread
½ whole wheat English muffin
½ whole wheat pita (6 in.)
¼ whole wheat bagel
½ whole wheat hamburger bun
1 small whole grain dinner roll
½ cup bran cereal
¾ cup unsweetened cereal
¼ cup low-sugar granola
½ cup oatmeal, plain
½ cup whole grain pasta, cooked
⅓ cup brown rice, cooked
⅓ cup whole wheat couscous, cooked
⅓ cup barley, cooked
½ cup bulgur, cooked
¼ cup spelt or kamut, cooked
3 Tbsp. wheat germ, dry
⅓ cup quinoa, cooked
½ cup corn
½ corn on the cob, large
½ cup green peas, cooked
½ cup mashed potatoes
½ baked/broiled potato, large
8-10 whole grain crackers
3 cups popcorn, plain

FRUITS (15 grams carbohydrate each)
Juice and fruit syrup should be avoided.
1 small apple, orange, peach
1 mini banana
4 apricots, fresh
1 Tbsp. raisins
¾ cup blueberries
1¼ cup strawberries
1 cup melon cubes or 1 slice
½ grapefruit, large
1 cup (about 12) grapes
2 plums
¾ cup pineapple
1 ¼ cup watermelon

MILK (12 grams carbohydrate)**
1 cup non-fat milk, any variety
6 oz. yogurt, plain or artificially sweetened

NON-STARCHY VEGGIES
(5 grams carbohydrate each)
½ cup cooked vegetables
1 cup raw vegetables

PROTEINS: (7 grams protein each)
Lean or low-fat are best. Consume several servings with all meals and snacks.*
1 oz. poultry, fish, beef, pork
1 whole egg
1 oz. cheese
½ cup (4 oz.) tofu
¼ cup ricotta/cottage cheese
1 oz. tuna
1 oz. shellfish
½ cup edamame (soybeans)

Exceptions:
1Tbsp. peanut butter = 1 protein, 2 fats
½ cup cooked beans = 1 protein, 1 starch
1 veggie burger, soy-based = 2 proteins

FATS: (5 grams fat each)
Avoid trans fats and limit saturated fats.*
1 tsp. oil
1 tsp. margarine/butter
1 tsp. regular mayo
1 Tbsp. cream cheese
1 slice bacon
2 Tbsp. half & half or cream
2 Tbsp. sour cream
1 Tbsp. salad dressing
1 Tbsp. sesame seeds
2 Tbsp. avocado
8 olives
10 peanuts
4 walnut halves
6 whole almonds
6 cashews
16 pistachios
2 tsp. peanut/almond butter
1 Tbsp. flax seed, ground

*These are approximate amounts. To find amounts for your specific needs consult with a registered dietitian.
**Although milk is a great protein source, it is also a source of carbohydrates.

Fruits contain carbohydrates. They also provide important vitamins, minerals, antioxidants and fiber that help prevent cancer and lower blood pressure, insulin and cholesterol. Because of their high fiber intake, eating fruit results in a slower release of sugar into your bloodstream (see Figure 2.0) and better insulin regulation.

All fruit in its natural, intact form is healthy and nutritious. Since each fruit has a different nutrient profile (bananas are high in potassium, oranges and kiwis high in vitamin C), eating a large variety is best. Fruit is easy to pack and very flavorful making them a great snack or an easy addition to a meal. However, like any carbohydrate, fruit should be eaten with caution. Eat it throughout the day and limit intake to one to two servings at meals and snacks. Fruit doesn't contain protein or fat, so you may want to eat it with protein or fat, such as nuts or cottage cheese, to increase satiety. Aim for three to five servings of fruit a day for maximum health. Fruit juice is very concentrated, lacks fiber and spikes insulin levels. Avoid it.

Remember all fruit is good for you. Portion size is the real culprit to weight gain. For example, bananas get a bad rap. Why the bad rap? Because people think they are high in sugar. The truth is that bananas are higher in sugar because they contain less water then most fruit; so one regular sized banana typically counts as two fruit servings. Buy baby bananas or cut one regular sized banana in half and save the rest for the next day's fruit servings, but don't avoid this amazing fruit because of its bad rap. Bananas have no fat, cholesterol or sodium. They are high in potassium, which regulates blood pressure, and they are a wonderful source of B vitamins, which help maintain blood sugar levels.

Think about your current fruit intake. How many servings do you get each day? A list of serving sizes is found in the PCOS Food Exchange List. _____

If you don't get the recommended amount of three to five servings each day, why? Do have any negative attitudes toward fruit? What can help you over come this?

_____

_____

_____

_____

_____

Here are some ideas to help incorporate more fruit into your diet. Circle or highlight the ones that appeal to you and add your own ideas to the list:

- Add fruit to oatmeal such as blueberries, cherries or bananas
- Grapes, apples and cranberries are great in a salad
- Snack on cottage cheese and your favorite fruit
- Add fruit such as mango or papaya to a smoothie
- Put apple slices on a sandwich
- Make a parfait out of plain non-fat yogurt, fruit and nuts
- Add peanut or almond butter to an apple
-
-
-

Vegetables, like fruit, provide numerous health benefits, thanks to their high fiber content and a rich supply of vitamins and nutrients. These benefits include improving blood pressure, cholesterol, insulin and preventing cancer. Just like fruit, the more variety, the better. There are two classifications of vegetables: Starchy and non-starchy. Starchy vegetables have a higher content of carbohydrates, similar to that of whole grains and fruits; they too need to be eaten with caution. As shown in Figure 2.0, starchy vegetables contribute to raising insulin levels more than non-starchy ones. Examples of starchy vegetables include corn, peas and potatoes and are listed under the Grains and Starches category in the PCOS Food Exchange List.

Foods like broccoli, zucchini, squash, spinach, green beans, onions and peppers are non-starchy vegetables and contribute little to increasing insulin levels. Non-starchy vegetables contain a lot of fiber and are low in calories, so you can eat them without caution to feel fuller and more satisfied with meals. Try to eat at least two to three non-starchy vegetable choices each day. In general, one non-starchy vegetable serving is a half cup of cooked vegetables, 1 cup of raw vegetables or 1 cup of vegetable juice.

Consider your vegetable intake. How many servings do you get each day? A list of serving sizes is found in the PCOS Food Exchange List. _____

If you don't get the recommended amount of three to five servings of vegetables each day, why? What steps could you take to increase your intake of vegetables? Do you have any negative attitudes toward vegetables? What can help you over come them?

_____

_____

Some ideas for adding more vegetables to your diet include:

- Adding chopped peppers, tomatoes or spinach to an omelet
- Include lettuce, tomato, pickles and onions on your sandwich

- Have low-sodium vegetable soups as part of a meal or as a snack
- Munch on baby carrots or celery dipped in hummus
- Add your favorite assorted vegetables to a garden salad
- Aim to cover half of your dinner plate with vegetables
- Top a slice of whole wheat pizza with vegetables

Legumes consist of lentils, beans and peas. Legumes provide a good source of plant-based proteins and are rich in fiber, folate, iron and other important vitamins and minerals. They are low in fat, have no cholesterol and are high in potassium and magnesium. Legumes are also an excellent source of protein, and like all vegetables, contain carbohydrates. When eating them in meals and snacks, you must balance (and account for) the carbohydrates in the legumes with other carbohydrate-containing foods. When consumed in moderation, legumes have a low impact on insulin levels (see Figure 2.0).

Ideas for incorporating legumes into your diet include:

- Adding chickpeas or black beans to salads
- Make a black bean dip to have with fresh cut up vegetables
- Add hummus to a sandwich or use it as a dip with vegetables
- Add your favorite beans to soups
- Have legumes as a side dish, such as a lentil salad, to your favorite meal

Milk is a rich source of calcium and protein, and is also considered a carbohydrate due to its high lactose content. Lactose is a natural sugar that is digested much slower than simple sugar or glucose. Although milk contains carbohydrates, drinking it results in a gradual release of glucose and insulin (see Figure 2.0).

Food labels don't differentiate sugar types (i.e., glucose or lactose). When you look at the nutrition label for milk, you will see 8 ounces of milk has approximately 12 grams of sugar. Since the sugar is lactose, don't be concerned about the sugar content for plain non-flavored milk. However, sugar content is a concern when choosing a milk-based product, like chocolate milk or flavored yogurt. You can tell where sugars have been added as they are listed in the ingredient list on the food label.

Milk is a rich source of carbohydrates and you will need to balance your intake with other carbohydrates you eat. For instance, instead of adding a glass of milk to a meal containing salmon (a protein) and corn (a carbohydrate), you may want to drink milk instead of eating corn or drink it with another meal that doesn't contain so many carbohydrates such as with an omelet and non-starchy vegetables. Drinking milk is also a great snack between meals, consumed cold or steamed with a sugar-free flavoring such as sugar-free vanilla.

Did you know that consuming dairy, especially full-fat types, may also improve your fertility? Interesting findings from the Nurses' Health Study[1] show that a daily serving or two of whole milk or whole-milk based products, such as full-fat yogurt, cheese, cottage cheese and even ice cream seem to offer some protection against ovulatory infertility (infertility caused by ovulation problems). Researchers still aren't sure why consuming a serving or two of full-fat dairy products improve fertility but speculate that skim and low-fat milk contain an imbalance of sex hormones that could affect ovulation and conception. Full-fat dairy products are high in calories and saturated fat, which increase risk of heart disease. Bottom line: If you are trying to get pregnant, you may want to consider temporarily consuming one or two servings a day of full-fat dairy products. Examples of a serving are 1 oz of cheese, 8 oz of whole milk, ¼ cup of cottage cheese or ½ cup of ice cream. Once you become pregnant or decide to stop trying, you may want to switch back to low-fat dairy products.

WHAT ABOUT PROTEIN?

Protein is essential. Protein foods mostly come from animal sources and include meat, poultry, pork, fish, seafood, eggs and dairy. Plant-based proteins include legumes (beans, lentils, peas), nuts and soy. Generally, proteins by themselves don't require much insulin to breakdown because protein doesn't get converted into glucose and doesn't raise insulin levels like carbohydrates (see Figure 2.0).

When the connection between PCOS and insulin resistance was first established in the mid-1990s, many health care professionals recommended women with PCOS eat a high protein and very low carbohydrate diet (under 100 grams of total carbohydrates per day). High protein/very low carbohydrate diets were probably believed to be superior to other diets in improving insulin resistance and weight loss because proteins don't increase insulin levels to the degree that carbohydrates do. This combined with the recent "no carb" diet rage may cause women with PCOS to fear carbs.

There are, however, many disadvantages to high protein diets for women with PCOS. High protein diets contain significant amounts of saturated fat and cholesterol because the proteins are typically animal products. As a result, high protein diets may put women with PCOS at a higher risk for heart disease and diabetes, especially since high protein diets restrict fruits, starchy vegetables and whole grains. Most people are unable to follow this diet for a long time because it severely limits carbs. Women with PCOS may have a particularly harder time following the diet because they have strong cravings for bread products and sweets. Carbohydrate deprivation often leads to overeating and weight gain, worsening PCOS. If you've tried a high protein/very low carbohydrate diet before, you know what I'm talking about!

---

1 The Nurses' Health Study, started in 1976 is one of the largest investigations to examine health habits and their affect on developing chronic diseases in over 120,000 nurses. In this particular study, researchers examined the eating habits of over 18,000 nurses from The Nurses' Health Study to investigate connections between diet and fertility. To learn more about The Nurses' Health Study, visit www.nurseshealthstudy.org.

The belief that women with PCOS need to adopt a high protein/very low carbohydrate diet is false. Numerous studies have examined the effects of high protein vs. low protein diets in women with PCOS. In one study, two groups of overweight women with PCOS were asked to follow either a high protein or low protein diet, each diet containing the same caloric content (1400 calories) for three months. Both groups showed similar results in lowering insulin and testosterone levels and improving weight loss and menstrual function. While studies show that weight loss is beneficial to improving PCOS, following a high protein and very low carbohydrate diet alone does not improve PCOS any more than a low protein and moderate carbohydrate diet. There is no reason for women with PCOS to severely limit their carbohydrate intake and follow a high protein diet for weight loss and improvement of symptoms.

Too much protein may also affect your fertility. Participants in the Nurses' Health Study were divided into groups depending on protein intake. After factoring in smoking, fat intake, weight and other variables that can affect fertility, researchers found that women in the highest-protein group were 41% more likely to report problems with ovulatory infertility (infertility caused by problems with ovulation) than women in the lowest-protein group.

Not only the amount, but the type of protein also matters. Women with the highest intake of meat had 39% more ovulatory infertility than those with the lowest meat intake. Those who consumed the most plant-based proteins had the lowest amount of infertility. The exceptions were eggs, dairy and fish, which were found to increase fertility.

Protein is essential for life. It gives us energy, maintains our muscles and best of all, adds to satiety which, in women with PCOS, helps prevent binges and low blood sugar. Instead of eating a diet high in protein and low in carbohydrates, your best bet is to stick with moderate amounts of proteins and carbohydrates. The PCOS Food Exchange List shows examples of popular proteins. Lean or low-fat proteins like low-fat cheese, tofu, fish, eggs, lean meats and chicken without the skin will fill you up without a lot of calories, saturated fat or cholesterol. You will need several servings (3 to 6 ounces) of lean protein at each meal or snack to feel satisfied and prevent low blood sugar. To give you an idea, 3 ounces is usually the size of a deck of cards or the palm of your hand (not including your fingers). If you are interested in learning more about your body's specific protein needs, consult a registered dietitian.

FAT FACTS

You may be wondering how fat fits into a healthy meal plan for PCOS. The good news: Dietary fat doesn't require insulin because it doesn't break down into glucose. The right types of fat used carefully in a healthy eating plan helps to improve insulin levels. The bad news: Dietary fat can affect insulin levels. You can't eat as much as you want. Diets high in saturated and trans fats contribute to insulin resistance and are the main contributors to high triglycerides and cholesterol. On the other hand, diets that contain too little fat may contribute to infertility as the majority of our sex hormones are controlled by dietary fat.

However, fat contains double the calories per gram compared to carbohydrates or protein, so moderation is needed.

WHY WE NEED FAT

Fat gets a bad rap, but you need it. It keeps us satisfied longer and prevents overeating. Dietary fats also provide a unique mouth feel and palatability to meals that carbohydrates and proteins do not. Diets containing too little fat can contribute to overeating or bingeing since they make you feel hungrier and less satisfied. Eating some fat with a meal or snack slows the release of glucose, resulting in a lower glycemic-index and better insulin management (see Figure 2.0).

SATURATED AND TRANS FAT

Why do you hear so much about saturated and trans fats? Because saturated fat contributes to insulin resistance and elevates cholesterol and triglycerides. Saturated fats, typically solid at room temperature, are found in animal products such as butter, cheese, luncheon meats, red meat, sour cream and mayonnaise. Certain oils, like palm kernel oil, are also saturated. These types of foods should be eaten sparingly. National dietary guidelines recommend that your saturated fat intake be no more than 10% of your total calorie intake. If you eat 1,800 calories a day, you should consume less than 20 grams of saturated fat.

Trans fats were initially created by food manufacturing companies to extend the shelf life of food and provide a unique texture and mouth feel. Trans fats are essentially the result of changing the chemical structure of a liquid fat into a solid fat. Trans fats raise LDL (the "bad") cholesterol and lower protective HDL (the "good" cholesterol). The amount of trans fats are listed on the Nutrition Facts panel so pay attention. However, just because a food claims to be trans fat-free does not mean it is healthy. Many manufacturers eliminated trans fats from their products then added saturated fats like palm kernel oil and other tropical oils. Products with 0.5 grams or less of trans fat per serving, can be listed as having zero grams of trans fat or trans fat-free. Also, any food containing shortening, partially or hydrogenated vegetable oil, interesterified or stearate-rich oil contains trans fats and should be avoided in your diet. Fast foods, chips, crackers, baked goods, cereals, candy and energy bars typically contain saturated and trans fats.

BENEFITS OF OMEGA-3 FATS

Not all fats are created equal. You may have heard about a class of fats called omega-3 fatty acids. There are three different types of omega-3 fats:

- alpha-linolenic acid (ALA) are plant based omega-3s found in walnuts, flaxseed, hemp and canola oil;
- eicosapentaenoic acid (EPA) and docosahexaenoic acid (DHA) are omega-3 fats

found in egg yolks and fatty or "oily" coldwater fish such as salmon, tuna, trout and halibut. Few other fish are rich in omega-3s.

Omega-3 fats are essential for women with PCOS. They help improve mood, decrease cholesterol and triglycerides, improve insulin, lower blood pressure and provide better hair and skin quality. Despite the benefits of omega-3 fatty acids, most Americans don't consume enough of them. This can be attributed to two main factors: Our diets lack foods rich in omega-3s or our diet is abundant in omega-6 fatty acids, which hamper the benefits of omega-3s. Omega-3 foods containing ALA get converted slowly into DHA and EPA in the body. For this reason, fish and fish oil are the preferred ways to meet optimal omega-3 intake.

Bottom line: Even if you eat fatty fish at least twice a week you should take a daily fish oil supplement consisting of 1 gram (1,000 mg) of a combination of EPA and DHA, not to exceed 4 grams (4,000 mg) daily. If you have high cholesterol or triglycerides, discuss how much omega-3s you need with your physician, especially if you are taking blood thinning medications. If you are vegetarian or vegan, you can take flaxseed oil which contains a rich amount of ALA.

The following are tips for incorporating omega-3 fats into your diet. Circle or highlight the ideas that may work for you. Can you add some others?

- Use canola oil in cooking and baking
- Add walnuts or sunflower seeds to salads
- Snack on walnuts alone or in a trail mix
- Stir ground flaxseed into cereal, oatmeal, yogurt or smoothies
- Grill a fatty type of fish (tuna, salmon, trout) and add to salads
- Prepare fatty fish and poultry with crushed almonds
- Take a fish oil supplement of at least 1 gram daily
- Eat eggs for breakfast or add to salads

Omega-6 fats

Having the right balance of fatty acids is essential for treatment, prevention and maintenance of inflammation, so commonly found in PCOS. Omega-6 fatty acids are unsaturated fats found in vegetable oils such as palm, soybean, corn, safflower, cottonseed, grapeseed and sunflower oil. These types of fats have flooded our food supply and are in most of the foods we eat. Excessive intake of omega-6 fats is associated with heart attacks, stroke, arrhythmia, arthritis, osteoporosis, inflammation, mood disorders and certain types of cancer.

The optimal ratio of omega-6 to omega-3 fats is 4 to 1. Most diets have ratios exceeding 10 to 1. Women with PCOS need to decrease foods they eat containing omega-6 fats and increase their intake of omega-3 fats to reap the benefits of omega-3s. Omega-6 fats are in margarine, some meats and poultry, baked goods, breads, crackers and salad dressings. You can spot them by checking the ingredient list. If palm, soybean, corn, safflower, cottonseed, grapeseed or sunflower oil are ingredients listed in your food, they contain omega-6 fats and should be limited.

Do you know which foods you eat contain omega-6 fats? Look at the ingredient list of your most commonly eaten foods. Pay close attention to salad dressings, baked goods and margarines. Write down the foods you eat that are sources of omega-6 fats:

_____   _____

_____   _____

_____   _____

_____   _____

_____   _____

How can you limit these foods?

_____

_____

_____

Mix it up!

If possible, include protein (ideally lean or low-fat) or fat (mostly omega-3 fats) in all your meals and snacks. Small meals and light snacks, about every 3 to 5 hours will satisfy you more, reduce cravings for carbohydrates and prevent low blood sugar. Tips for healthy snacking can be found in the next chapter or come up with your own ideas by using the PCOS Food Exchange List. Experiment with different food combinations to see what foods satisfy you the most.

Name some protein-rich snacks or meals that work well for you and keep you satisfied:

_____   _____

_____   _____

_____   _____

_____   _____

Summary of Recommended Nutrition Guidelines for PCOS:

- Consume a variety of foods from all food groups
- Avoid sweetened beverages
- Eat every 3 to 5 hours
- Eat carbohydrate-containing foods evenly throughout the day
- Eliminate refined carbohydrates and simple sugars
- Consume lean protein sources or foods rich in omega-3 fats with all meals or snacks
- Eliminate trans and saturated fats and limit foods containing omega-6 fats
- Consume fatty fish (trout, salmon, halibut, tuna) twice a week and/or take at least 1 gram of fish oil daily

Remember, the main treatment goal for PCOS is to reduce insulin levels. In this chapter, we discussed how food affects insulin levels and how you can best manage your insulin levels with food. Now that you are better informed about foods that contribute to insulin resistance (simple and refined carbohydrates) and which foods can improve insulin resistance (balance of whole grains, lean proteins, fruits, vegetables and omega-3 fats) you can make better choices to improve your health. In the next two chapters, we will discuss some ways to take control of your food selection and examine what gets in the way of you making better food choices.

CHAPTER 3

NUTRITION 411

THIS chapter will give you the 411 on nutrition and exercise for PCOS. In the previous chapter, we discussed how food affects your insulin levels. This chapter teaches you how to read food labels, helps you make smart food choices and offers tips for eating out and healthy snacking. In addition, we'll discuss some of the best nutrition supplements you should take to improve your PCOS.

PCOS NUTRITION QUIZ

Before we begin learning about nutrition for PCOS, take a moment to assess your nutrition knowledge and attitudes by taking this quiz. Answers are found at the end of this chapter.

True or False

1. _____ I have to eat very low-carb to lose weight.

2. _____ Whole grain foods contain fiber.

3. _____ Physical activity will improve my insulin levels.

4. _____ Certain dietary supplements can improve PCOS.

5. _____ Binge eating is common in women with PCOS.

6. _____ Women with PCOS shouldn't eat fruit.

7. _____ If I lift weights I will get bigger and bulkier.

8. _____ I have to lose a lot of weight to improve my health.

9. _____ Tilapia is a fish rich in omega-3 fatty acids.

10. _____ An item labeled "100% wheat" is a whole grain food.

THE WHOLE TRUTH: SHOPPING FOR WHOLE GRAINS AND READING FOOD LABELS

Have you become more aware of shopping for whole grains? Most consumers are recognizing the benefits of whole grain foods in their diet. In fact, manufacturers are capitalizing on the renewed interest by using clever marketing strategies to lure consumers into buying their products. Don't be fooled. Some manufacturers use coloring agents to give their products a whole grain "look." You must read labels. Just because a food looks whole grain, says "high fiber" or "multigrain" on the package, doesn't mean it's a whole grain product. If the first item on the ingredient list doesn't say "whole," it's not a whole grain product (see Figure 3.0 for examples). If a food is labeled "stone-ground," "wheat flour," "100% wheat," "seven-grain," or "bran" it's not necessarily a whole grain product. Figure 3.1 shows the ingredient list of a whole grain food. A list of examples of whole grain foods is shown in Figure 3.2.

Figure 3.0. Examples of first ingredients *not* indicating whole grain.

Enriched wheat flour
Wheat
Multigrain
Wheat flour
Seven-grain blend
Brown rice syrup

Figure 3.1. A whole grain food as shown on an ingredient list.

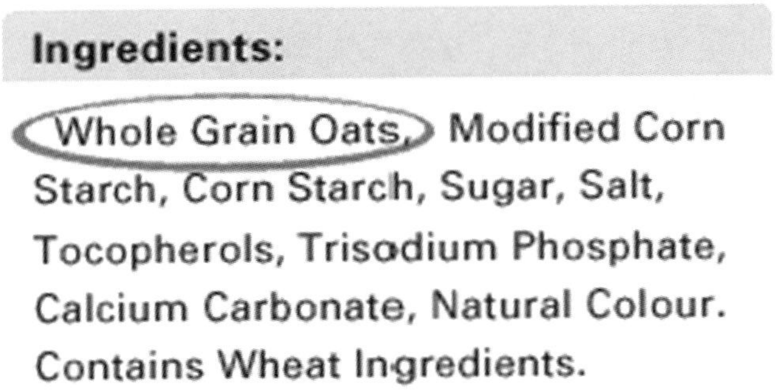

Ingredients:

Whole Grain Oats, Modified Corn Starch, Corn Starch, Sugar, Salt, Tocopherols, Trisodium Phosphate, Calcium Carbonate, Natural Colour. Contains Wheat Ingredients.

This food is a whole grain food. Note that the first ingredient says 'whole.'

Figure 3.2. Examples of first ingredients indicating whole grain.

> Whole wheat
> Whole grain
> Whole wheat flour
> Bulgur
> Whole oats
> Whole rye
> Wild or brown rice
> Stone-ground whole wheat flour

The non-profit Whole Grains Council (www.wholegrainscouncil.org) has developed a Whole Grain Stamp indicating when a food is mostly whole grain. The stamp is now displayed on more than 900 products. Distinctive with a black and gold print, the Whole Grain stamp is easy to identify on packages. As shown in Figure 3.3, each stamp displays the number of grams of whole grains in a serving. To qualify for the stamp, each product serving must provide at least a half-serving (eight grams) or more of whole grain. Foods in which all grains are whole (no refined grain added) are listed as 100% whole grain.

Figure 3.3. Examples of the whole grain stamp.

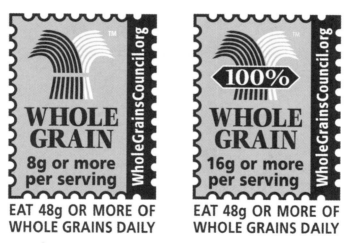

Courtesy of Oldways and the Whole Grains Council

Just because a food is whole grain doesn't mean it's healthy. You must look at sugar content. The amount of sugar is shown on a food label listed under carbohydrates (see Figure 3.4). If a food item says a serving has 30 grams of total carbohydrates and 25 grams of sugar, most of those carbs are sugar, not whole grains. A good example: Flavored instant oatmeal. It is a whole grain (first ingredient is whole oats) but the flavoring adds sugar, resulting in a high glycemic-index, that will increase your insulin levels. Be sure to eat only plain or sugar-free flavored oatmeal.

Take a look at this Nutrition Facts Panel (Figure 3.4). A half cup of this food has 32 grams of total carbohydrates and has 18 grams of sugar. This means almost half of the carbohydrates are sugar. Eating this food will spike insulin levels.

Figure 3.4. An example of a high sugar food.

Nutrition Facts
Serving Size 1/2 cup (57g)
Servings Per Container 15

Amount Per Serving

Calories 230   Calories from Fat 100

	% Daily Value*
Total Fat 11g	17%
Saturated Fat 2g	10%
Trans Fat 0g	
Cholesterol 0mg	0%
Sodium 95mg	4%
Total Carbohydrate 32g	11%
Dietary Fiber 3g	12%
Sugars 18g	
Protein 5g	

Vitamin A 0% • Vitamin C 0%

Calcium 4% • Iron 10%

*Percent Daily Values are based on a 2,000 calorie diet. Your daily values may be higher or lower depending on your calorie needs:

		Calories 2,000	2,500
Total Fat	Less Than	65g	80g
Saturated Fat	Less Than	20g	25g
Cholesterol	Less Than	300mg	300 mg
Sodium	Less Than	2,400mg	2,400mg
Total Carbohydrate		300g	375g
Dietary Fiber		25g	30g

Calories per gram:
Fat 9 • Carbohydrate 4 • Protein 4

Grocery shopping in America can be overwhelming. Never has one country had so many food options. New foods are introduced almost daily. The bread isle alone can extend the entire length of the store! There are numerous types and brands of white, rye, pumpernickel and wheat breads, all with various ingredients and claims. Do you get overwhelmed with all the choices? You're not alone. When choosing a food, ask yourself the following three questions:

1. Does the first ingredient say 'whole'?
2. Does the food have more grams of fiber than its counterparts?
3. Does the food have the least amount of sugar compared to its counterparts?

If you can answer "yes" to all three, buy it. Check out this great website for reading labels: www.labelwatch.com.

LIFE BEYOND WHEAT

Now that you know the role whole grains play in a healthy PCOS diet, here's how to incorporate them into your diet. The following information introduces different types of whole grains and how you can use them. For specific recipes, check out these websites: www.epicurious.com, www.cookinglight.com, wholegrainscouncil.org and www.wheatfoods.org. Some grains are used in the sample menu plans found in the appendix.

Amaranth. A staple of the Incas and the Aztecs, amaranth is a tiny yellowish-brown grain that packs a hefty nutritional profile. Its seeds have more protein, iron, potassium, phosphorous, calcium and magnesium than any other grain. In addition, its naturally occurring amino acids, lysine, methionine and cysteine, are limited in other grains. Amaranth has a nutty flavor, especially when it is toasted before grinding. The seeds can be used in breads or popped like popcorn then eaten as a snack.

Bulgur. Also referred to as cracked wheat, bulgur is considered a pseudograin that begins as a whole wheat kernel, then is boiled, dried and cracked into small pieces, removing 5% of the bran. It's a staple in Middle Easterners' diets and is the main ingredient in tabouli. Bulgur has a nutty, chewy texture and easy to prepare as it doesn't need to be washed before cooking. Bulgur swells during cooking, requiring an adequate sized pot and can be cooked in the microwave or on stovetop. It can be used in meatloafs, soups, stews, casseroles and baked goods.

Flaxseed. Cultivated as early as 3,000 B.C., flaxseed is now a household name and for good reason! Flaxseed provides protein, vitamins, minerals, soluble and insoluble fiber, phytoestrogens, and is an excellent source of essential fatty acids. Flaxseeds are best digested when ground (use a coffee grinder) and should be stored in an airtight container in the refrigerator. Flaxseed can be sprinkled in cereal, oatmeal, soups and yogurt or used in breads, muffins or crackers. When baking, milled flaxseed can be substituted for shortening, oils or eggs (for every egg being replaced, mix 1 tablespoon of milled flax with 3 tablespoons water).

Kamut. Kamut, an ancient Egyptian word that means wheat, has a buttery, nutty flavor and is a close relative to durum. It contains eight amino acids, which gives the grain one of the highest protein contents among grains. It is also rich in vitamin E and B vitamins. Kamut is mostly found in bread products such as cereals, crackers and pasta.

Millet. There are more than 6,000 varieties of millet. Its tiny, round and yellow kernels contain high amounts of protein, B vitamins, vitamin E, calcium, iron and phosphorous plus its oil is unsaturated. Millet contains more calories than wheat because of its higher oil content. Millet has a similar texture to wild rice and has a mild flavor that makes it very versatile. It can be used as an ingredient in side dishes, such as rice pilaf and stuffing, or used as porridge.

Quinoa. Pronounced KEEN-wa, quinoa is the powerhouse of grains and has quickly risen in popularity due to its excellent nutrition profile, texture and ease of use. Quinoa seeds are small, flat and rounded, similar to that of sesame seeds. Quinoa has a nutty taste with a soft, crunchy texture. Quinoa provides all essential amino acids, making it a complete protein, and has approximately twice the protein as regular grains. Rich in B vitamins, vitamin A, magnesium, phosphorous, iron, fiber and calcium, this food is relatively high in unsaturated fat. Quinoa is technically not a grain but a fruit and is a great alternative to couscous or rice. Use quinoa to make pilafs, risottos, stews, salads or even desserts. Quinoa can also serves as an excellent high-protein breakfast served hot, mixed with berries, nuts or cinnamon. Rinse well prior to cooking to remove its bitter waxy protective coating.

Spelt. Spelt is rich in B vitamins and contains eight essential amino acids. Spelt has a sweet and nutty taste with a chewy texture. Used as a slow-cooked grain, use spelt in soups and stews, like barley, or substituted in recipes calling for rice. Spelt can also be used as an ingredient in cookies, quick breads and muffins.

Tips To Add Whole Grain Foods To Your Diet

- Include a whole grain cereal, quinoa or plain oatmeal with breakfast or snacks
- Add whole grains to dishes, such as barley, in vegetable soup and stews or add prepared bulgur or flaxseed to waffles, pancakes, muffins or baked goods for a nutty flavor
- Make sandwiches with whole grain bread
- Substitute whole grain pastas for regular pasta
- Try quick-cooking versions of brown rice, barley and whole wheat couscous as side dishes to meals
- Use rolled oats or a crushed whole grain cereal to coat chicken, fish or veal
- Snack on whole grain crackers or air-popped popcorn

Write down examples of whole grains that you would like to try and ideas on how you can incorporate them:

_____

_____

_____

_____

PASS THE PLANT STEROLS PLEASE!

Have you ever heard of plant sterols or stanols? Naturally found in vegetable oils, nuts and whole grains, plant sterols are now being added to numerous foods like juice, granola bars, mayonnaise, margarines, milk and even multi-vitamins. Adding plant sterols to your diet is one of the simplest ways to lower your cholesterol. Plant sterols have the same structure as cholesterol and interfere with its absorption. The National Cholesterol Education Program recommends you consume 2 grams of plant sterols per day if you have elevated cholesterol. Figure 3.5 show sources of plant sterols along with amounts. Be sure to look for plant sterols on food labels when shopping.

Figure 3.5. **Food sources of plant sterols.**

Avocados, 1 small	0.13 grams
Corn Oil, 1 tablespoon	0.13 grams
Sunflower Seeds, 1/4 cup	0.19 grams
Oat Bar with plant sterols, 1 bar	0.4 grams
Orange Juice, 1 cup with plant sterols	1.0 gram
Vegetable oil spread with plant sterols, 1 tablespoon	1.0 gram
Fruit & yogurt flavored drink with plant sterols, 3 oz. bottle	2.0 grams

TIPS FOR EATING OUT

Who doesn't enjoy eating out? Sitting and relaxing while being served good food is a luxury we often take for granted. However, having PCOS and dining out can pose some challenges. Large portions and that constant presence of the bread basket (with butter or oil!) at the center of the table pose two of the biggest challenges. Dining out and eating is tough, but not impossible. Be smart about your food selections, portion size, listen to your body and stop when you feel yourself getting full. Below are some exercises and tips to help you enjoy your meal while still following the nutrition guidelines for PCOS.

Take a few minutes to think about the most difficult challenges you face when dining out? What is difficult? Write them here:

_____

_____

_____

_____

The plate method

Follow the steps below to get a sense of what your plate should look like. This can be helpful when you eat out or are preparing your meals at home.

1. In the space provided, draw a large circle to represent your dinner or lunch plate.
2. Draw a line straight through the middle of it.
3. Starting on the right side, draw a line straight through the middle to separate it into quarters.
4. On the left half of your plate, write 'Non-starchy Vegetables'.
5. In one of the open quarters write the word 'Protein'.
6. In the remaining quarter write 'Whole Grain Starches'.

What do you notice about your plate? Does it look awkward or foreign? Do you typically eat like this? What if this was your actual plate?

_____

_____

_____

_____

_____

More tips for eating out

- **Be prepared.** If you know the restaurant in advance, take time to think about food choices and what you plan to order. Many restaurants post their menus online.
- **Say 'No' to the bread basket.** If you know you will be having several carbohydrates, consider passing on the bread basket. Refuse it altogether or take a piece and ask that the rest be removed.
- **Be mindful.** Check in with yourself when you first sit down. Do some deep breathing. Ask yourself to rate how hungry you are from a scale of 1 to 10 (1 not hungry and 10 stuffed). Do this again in the middle of your meal. Practice recognizing when you are getting satisfied and stop eating.
- **Wrap it up.** When satisfied, ask that your food be removed or wrapped up. Place your utensils down on your plate to signal to yourself and your server that you are done eating.
- **Avoid saboteurs.** Do you have a friend or partner who sabotages your eating? Maybe he or she encourages you to order a not-so-healthy entrée or appetizer? Have a game plan ahead of time to handle this. Will talking to the person beforehand help? Will choosing a different restaurant help?

Write down suggestions and strategies to help you deal with the challenges of dining out. In the past, what has helped and what hasn't, and why?

_____

_____

_____

SMART SNACKING

One of the most common questions asked by clients with PCOS is "what else can I eat for snacks?" Many of us are in a snack rut, eating the same snacks and not feeling particularly satisfied. This often leads to a vending machine run or a trip to the break room where less-nutritious foods are available.

Women with PCOS need to eat often throughout the day. Eating often will decrease cravings and prevent binges, provide energy and help prevent low blood sugar. Women with PCOS should eat every three to five hours and include a lean protein and/or fat with each meal or snack.

Preparation is key to making successful food choices, but it doesn't have to be difficult. If you know you get hungry in the afternoon or come home ravenous, plan for those times. On Monday, try bringing in enough snacks for the whole week, that way you don't have to be bogged down with yet another thing to remember. Spend some time on the weekend washing and cutting up vegetables and fruit, putting them in individual plastic bags or containers in appropriate portion-sizes. Or, pack snacks for the next day while making dinner. Have plenty of packing materials on hand, like sandwich bags, plastic wrap, foil and glass or plastic containers.

Here are some healthy snack suggestions. Can you add other ideas?

- Fruit and low-fat cheese
- Apple or celery and peanut butter
- Low-fat cottage cheese and fruit
- Non-fat, low sugar yogurt with ground flaxseed
- Hardboiled eggs
- Plain oatmeal and walnuts
- Latte with non-fat milk
- Trail mix of nuts, dried fruit and dark chocolate
- Whole wheat crackers with low-fat cheese or peanut butter
- Pomegranate seeds
- Wasabi dried peas
- Whole wheat fig bars
- High protein, whole grain and low-sugar bars
- Instant low-sodium bean or vegetable soups
- Whole grain pretzels
- Raw nuts such as walnuts and almonds
- Single-serving pouches of tuna
- Dark chocolate (at least 60% coco or higher. Limit to one to two squares)
- Mixed fruit cup
- Hummus and vegetables
- Edamame
-
-
-

Some final tips: Remember that food portions matter and be sure to vary your snacks to prevent boredom and maximize your nutritional intake. High-fiber foods, such as fruits, vegetables and whole grains, will make you fuller and can help keep you satisfied longer.

A WORD ON SODIUM

Almost all Americans consume too much sodium. Sodium is found in fast food and processed foods (canned, frozen and boxed items), meats and cheeses. The amount of sodium in food is listed in The Nutrition Facts panel on the package (see Figure 3.4). Government guidelines suggest we consume less than 2,400 mg of sodium per day. To give you an idea, just 1 teaspoon of salt has 2,000 mg!

Too much sodium raises your blood pressure. To decrease sodium in your diet, try choosing reduced or low-sodium products and don't pick up the salt shaker to flavor food. Instead, flavor foods with olive oil, herbs, spices or lemon. If you have high blood pressure, cut back on sodium and increase your intake of fruits and vegetables to help lower blood pressure.

Go through your kitchen cabinets, freezer, and refrigerator and look at sodium amounts in your foods. Sodium is listed in grams on the food label. Write down some of the foods you find that are high in sodium and record the amounts here:

Food item   Amount of sodium (in grams)

_____   _____

_____   _____

_____   _____

_____   _____

_____   _____

_____   _____

What can you do to reduce your intake of high sodium foods? Can you choose lower sodium versions or limit how much you eat? Write down at least one thing you can do to reduce your intake of sodium:

_____

_____

_____

_____

It's time for a meal makeover!

You've been given lots of eating tips and guidelines in this workbook. In the space below, write out a sample day of eating. Pick meals that are appealing and satisfying to you. Remember you need to eat every three to five hours and include some form of lean protein or healthy fat with each meal and snack. Fill in snacks if and when you will need them. Don't forget to write in the times you eat and indicate if a food is whole grain or not. Also be sure to identify portion sizes.

Sample Day

Breakfast (Time:)

Snack   **(Time:)**

Lunch   **(Time:)**

Snack   **(Time:)**

Dinner   **(Time:)**

Snack   **(Time:)**

How did it feel to do this exercise? Was it difficult or easy?

_____

_____

_____

_____

How realistic is it for you to follow what you planned? How does this sample day compare to how you currently eat? Do you think you could write out your meal plans on a daily basis? Why or why not?

_____

_____

_____

_____

_____

THE SCOOP ON NUTRITION SUPPLEMENTS

According to the National Institutes of Health (NIH) Office of Dietary Supplements, consumers spent $20.3 billion on dietary supplements in 2004. The NIH attributes this trend to several factors including increased availability of supplements, desire for control of one's own destiny, perception of increased safety and disillusionment with traditional medicine. If you are like many women with PCOS — who have been misdiagnosed, have not seen improvement in symptoms and are frustrated with your medical care — you may have considered or tried alternative treatments in hopes of getting better results.

Currently, supplements are not fully regulated by the Food and Drug Administration (FDA). Taking supplements alone or with medications poses risks. Supplements and drugs utilize the same metabolic pathway in the liver, increasing the chances for an interaction that could alter the effect of the supplement or medication possibly resulting in serious side effects, even death. Many women with PCOS do not tell their physicians which dietary or herbal supplements they are taking. Inform your doctor or health professional if you take any nutritional supplements.

Write down all the supplements (with amounts) you take. If you take a multivitamin, write the amounts of each supplement as listed on the label. Some labels will list potential risks or interactions with medications. Write down these risks or interactions here:

Name of supplement	Amount	Potential risk/interaction

The following supplements help lessen PCOS symptoms with the least side effects. For best results, take these supplements everyday.

Vitamin D. Did you know that vitamin D is not only a vitamin but also a hormone? Vitamin D receptors have been identified in almost every tissue and cell in the human body. It plays a part in follicle egg maturation and development as well as glucose regulation, notably in decreasing insulin resistance. Studies have shown that the majority of individuals in the United States are deficient in vitamin D. Low levels of vitamin D have been found in individuals with type 1 and type 2 diabetes. Few foods other than milk, eggs, liver, cereals with vitamin D added and fatty fish contain vitamin D. Skin exposure to sunlight provides as much as 80% to 90% of the body's vitamin D. However, overweight individuals have a greater chance of being deficient because vitamin D is a fat-soluble vitamin stored in high amounts of fatty tissue. All women with PCOS should take at least 1,000 IU of vitamin D daily and have your doctor check your vitamin D levels.

Cinnamon. Research indicates that cinnamon may help better regulate insulin levels and lower cholesterol. Side effects are very minimal, if any. Cinnamon lowers blood sugar so if you have diabetes and take cinnamon, careful monitoring of your blood sugar is important. This spice contains no calories or carbohydrates, making it an easy way to add it to your diet. Sprinkle it on cereal, coffee drinks, peanut butter sandwiches, oatmeal, cottage cheese, yogurt and many other foods. It can also be taken in a capsule form sold as cinnamon cassia extract to meet therapeutic dosages of 3 to 6 grams daily or 1 to 2 teaspoons daily.

Inositol. Inositol is a component of the cell membrane. Women with PCOS may try taking this supplement to decrease triglyceride and testosterone levels, and reduce high blood pressure. Inositol may also improve ovulation by improving insulin sensitivity. Generally, it's well tolerated but can cause nausea, fatigue, headaches and dizziness. No interactions with herbs and supplements are known. There is concern, however, that high consumption of inositol might exacerbate bipolar disorder. Dosage is 2,000 to 4,000 mg daily.

Fish oil. A fish oil supplement is a concentrated mix of different omega-3 fatty acids (EPA and DHA) found in fish. Research indicates fish oil is effective at improving all aspects of PCOS including insulin, triglycerides, blood pressure, cholesterol, mood and skin. DHA is particularly important during pregnancy as it aids in baby's brain development.

Dietary guidelines recommend that we consume cold water or oily fish two times per week to reap the benefits of omega-3 fatty acids found in fish. Salmon, halibut, tuna and trout are the best sources of omega-3s. Even if you eat oily fish twice a week or more, you should consider taking a fish oil supplement. You can purchase fish oil in a gel capsule or a liquid form. Women with PCOS should take 1 to 4 grams daily. Talk to your physician before taking these supplements, especially if you take blood thinning medications. Side effects are minimal but include heartburn and burping. You can freeze gel capsules to decrease these effects.

Magnesium. Magnesium is found in certain types of fish, whole grains, fruits and vegetables, nuts, seeds, legumes and soy products. It has been suggested that women with PCOS have low magnesium levels. Magnesium supplementation may be beneficial to women with PCOS due to its ability to reduce insulin, glucose, cholesterol, blood pressure and overall risk of metabolic syndrome. Approximately 600 mg daily is needed to see results. Side effects are rare.

Now that we have reviewed some of the most beneficial supplements for improving PCOS, which are you are most interested in trying? What other information do you need to know before you take them?

_____

_____

_____

_____

_____

This is just a small list of nutritional supplements that may help improve your symptoms. Have you heard about others that weren't discussed here? If so, write them down:

_____

_____

_____

_____

_____

Hopefully this chapter gave you the information you need to make healthier food choices. If the information feels overwhelming, incorporate changes slowly instead of all at once. Maybe start with the suggestions that seem most doable to you. Remember, any changes you make and sustain will result in long-term improvements in your PCOS and your health.

ANSWERS: PCOS NUTRITION QUIZ

1. I have to eat very low-carb to lose weight. **False**. There is no evidence suggesting that low-carbohydrate diets are more beneficial at weight loss for PCOS than any other diet compositions. Low-carbohydrate diets lead to constipation, extreme fatigue and binge eating. Although you can lose weight on these diets, rarely are low-carbohydrate diets followed long-term resulting in weight gain once you stop the diet.

2. Whole grain foods contain fiber. **True**. High fiber foods, like whole grains have many health benefits, including lowering cholesterol and insulin levels, adding fullness to meals and maintaining your digestive system. Since whole grains are just that - a whole grain, all its layers are intact, including the layers that contain the fiber. For a food to be considered truly whole grain it must have the word 'whole' as part of the first ingredient in the ingredient list.

3. Physical activity will improve my insulin levels. **True**. Exercise, whether cardio, weight training or both, is very effective in decreasing insulin resistance.

4. Dietary supplements can improve PCOS. **True.** Some dietary supplements can improve insulin levels. Some of these supplements include vitamin D, chromium, cinnamon, fish oils and magnesium.

5. Binge eating is common for women with PCOS. **True.** Waiting too long to eat, combined with elevated insulin levels, hormone imbalances, negative body image and mood shifts put women with PCOS at higher risk for binge eating.

6. Women with PCOS shouldn't eat fruit. **False.** While fruit is a carbohydrate source, it contains many of the vitamins, minerals and fiber needed to improve insulin resistance and prevent the onset of cardiovascular disease and diabetes.

7. If I lift weights, I will get bigger and bulkier. **False.** While the general physique of a woman with PCOS is more masculine, this doesn't mean you will look like Arnold Schwarzenegger if you lift weights. Lifting weights is a great way to improve your insulin levels and without adding extra bulk.

8. I have to lose a lot of weight to improve my health. **False.** Dropping as little as 5% to 10% of your total body weight can significantly improve insulin levels and regulate menstrual cycles, as well as lower the risk of cardiovascular disease and diabetes in women with PCOS. This means if you weigh 220 pounds, you will greatly improve your health and fertility by losing between 11 and 22 pounds.

9. Tilapia is a fish rich in omega-3 fatty acids. **False.** While tilapia is one of the most common fish consumed, it is not a good source of omega-3 fats. Oily fish or cold water fish are rich in omega-3 fatty acids. These include salmon, tuna, halibut and trout.

10. A food labeled "100% wheat" is a whole grain food. **False.** It's not a whole grain because the word 'whole' isn't there. If it were a whole grain, it would read '100% whole wheat.'

CHAPTER 4

COMMITTING TO CHANGE: ANALYZING YOUR EATING AND EXERCISE PATTERNS

Do you really know what you eat or how often you are physically active? Remembering what you had for dinner last night can be a challenge let alone knowing what you ate all week. The purpose of this chapter is to help you take a close and honest look at your eating and physical activity habits. Awareness is the first step to making changes. Once you are aware of your habits and how well you meet the nutrition and exercise guidelines discussed in this book, you will have the opportunity to commit to setting goals related to your eating and/or exercise.

LET'S GET PHYSICAL!

Physical activity is one of the most effective treatments for PCOS. In fact, it is equally important as taking medications and a healthy diet. Both aerobic exercise (cardiovascular) and weight lifting can improve insulin levels. When our muscle cells get worked out, they're able to use insulin much more effectively. This means when we get moving, our bodies don't need to produce extra insulin. Exercising has also been shown to improve ovulation, either on its own or in combination with a healthy diet.

Benefits of Physical Activity

- Improves insulin sensitivity
- Helps weight management
- Improves ovulation
- Lowers stress
- Lowers blood pressure and cholesterol
- Contributes to a positive body image and mood

If you are like some women with PCOS, you may fear that lifting weights will contribute to a bigger and bulkier body. It's true that women with PCOS tend to have a more muscular shape, however, it's physically impossible for women to have the large, protruding muscles that men create by lifting weights. Consistency is key. Women with PCOS should engage in

30 to 60 minutes of daily physical activity. Taking a 10-minute walk in the morning, at lunch and in the evening is equally as effective as a 30-minute walk once a day. The key is to get your heart rate up and break a sweat. Want to know if you're heart rate is up high enough? Use the talk test: If it's difficult to maintain a conversation while exercising, your heart rate is up to the desired level. If you can't hold a conversation at all, you are working too hard.

People are more likely to stick with activities they enjoy. This could be gardening, playing tennis, biking, golfing, ballroom dancing or swimming instead of the typical stationary bike or treadmill. Maybe you enjoy group activities like water aerobics, pilates or a spinning class. If your unhappiness with your body is getting in the way of you doing regular movement, you need to get past this. Consider working with a therapist to challenge your negative body image.

Changing your lifestyle to accommodate more movement is one way to increase the amount of activity you do. You could: Take the stairs instead of the elevator, park your car further away from the store, carry a basket at the market instead of pushing a cart, get up and walk to a co-workers desk instead of emailing them. These ideas may not seem like much, but every little bit helps your body utilize insulin better. Some people are motivated by wearing a pedometer during the day. Try to reach 10,000 steps each day, the equivalent of about 5 miles. Not only will physical activity make you healthier but will help with your mood, stress, body image and self-esteem. There are no excuses not to move! Consult your physician before starting an exercise program.

What type of movement do you do each day? Do you clean your house, take the stairs instead of the elevator, park further away at the mall, play tennis or walk? List them here along with how each activity makes you feel:

_____

_____

_____

_____

_____

If you don't get regular physical activity, why? What excuses do you tell yourself? Are resources or support available to help overcome these barriers?

_____

_____

_____

_____

_____

What forms of movement do you like to do or wish you could learn to do? How can you fit these into your week?

_____

_____

_____

_____

_____

If you're already physically active, what helps you remain consistent with your activity? Do you challenge yourself to increase the intensity, variety or duration of your exercise?

_____

_____

_____

_____

_____

Are you willing to commit to adding more movement into your day and week? Goals could be simply agreeing to research an activity that appeals to you or be more specific such as "I will walk at lunch for 15 minutes each day," or "I will do water aerobics three times each week."

_____

_____

_____

_____

_____

WHAT ARE YOU EATING?

Now it's time for you to take an honest look at your food intake and eating habits. In the food records following, write everything (I mean everything!) you eat in the next three days. You want the record to reflect your normal patterns of eating. If you are about to go on vacation or are nearing a holiday, you may want to wait to start your record afterward. Keep a small notebook with you wherever you go and write down what you eat. When you get home, transfer the information into the logs provided. The PCOS Food Exchange List (found in Chapter 2 and in the appendix) can help you identify serving sizes and food categories. Don't forget to fill in where and when you ate the food, the time you ate and then rate how hungry you were before and how satisfied you were after you ate. Once you have entered all the information for three days and added up the total amounts for each food group, answer the questions that follow. Use the space below each question to write goals or ideas about how to change your eating patterns and improve your health. Chapter 7 will go into more detail about using food records to practice mindful eating and provide real-life examples.

How to use the food record

Time: Enter the time you ate.

Food eaten and amount: Estimate the amount of food you ate (e.g. ½ cup oatmeal, 1 apple, 1 oz. cheese) and use the PCOS Food Exchange List found in the appendix to determine how many servings of each food group you ate. For example, one apple = 1 fruit, 1 oz. cheese = 1 protein, or 2 slices of bread = 2 grains/starches. Don't forget to include beverages.

Hunger and Satisfaction Scale: Use this self-rating scale to determine how hungry you were before you ate and then rate how satisfied or full you were after your meal.

1. Completely empty. Beyond starving.
2. Very hungry. You need to eat now!
3. Getting pretty hungry and will need to eat very soon.
4. Starting to feel the urge to eat.
5. Neutral. Not hungry. Not full.
6. Starting to feel like the food is enough.
7. The food is enough. Stop here and you won't be hungry again for awhile.
8. Pretty full and starting to get uncomfortable.
9. Uncomfortable. Ate too much.
10. So completely stuffed that it's painful.

Place/thoughts/feelings/symptoms: Record where you ate the food, as well as any thoughts, feelings or emotions you experienced during the meal or any distorted eating symptoms that occurred (e.g. bingeing, purging, restricting).

Physical activity: Record the length and type of physical activity you did.

Time	Food Eaten & Amount	Grains / Starches	Protein	Fats	Fruits	Vegetables	Hunger / Satisfaction	Thoughts, feelings, symptoms
							1 2 3 4 5 6 7 8 9 10	
							1 2 3 4 5 6 7 8 9 10	
							1 2 3 4 5 6 7 8 9 10	
							1 2 3 4 5 6 7 8 9 10	
							1 2 3 4 5 6 7 8 9 10	
	Total Amount						Medication AM ☐ PM ☐	Physical Activity
	Recommended Amount							☐☐☐☐☐☐☐

Time	Food Eaten & Amount	Grains / Starches	Protein	Fats	Fruits	Vegetables	Hunger / Satisfaction	Thoughts, feelings, symptoms
							1 2 3 4 5 6 7 8 9 10	
							1 2 3 4 5 6 7 8 9 10	
							1 2 3 4 5 6 7 8 9 10	
							1 2 3 4 5 6 7 8 9 10	
							1 2 3 4 5 6 7 8 9 10	
Total Amount							Medication AM ☐ PM ☐	Physical Activity
Recommended Amount								

Time	Food Eaten & Amount	Grains / Starches	Protein	Fats	Fruits	Vegetables	Hunger / Satisfaction	Thoughts, feelings, symptoms
							1 2 3 4 5 6 7 8 9 10	
							1 2 3 4 5 6 7 8 9 10	
							1 2 3 4 5 6 7 8 9 10	
							1 2 3 4 5 6 7 8 9 10	
							1 2 3 4 5 6 7 8 9 10	

Total Amount / Recommended Amount

Medication AM☐ PM☐

Physical Activity

Copyright www.PCOSnutrition.com

1. Look at the time between your meals and snacks. Did you eat throughout the day, such as every three to five hours as suggested?

   If you answered yes, keep it up! Eating often will help prevent cravings and overeating as well as manage low blood sugar.

   If no, which meals have long periods of time between them?

   _____

   _____

   What can you do to eat more often during these times?

   _____

   _____

2. Review your food choices. Did you have protein and/or fat with your meals and snacks?

   If yes, you're more likely to feel satisfied longer and you are decreasing the glycemic response to carbohydrates. This will result in less insulin secretion.

   If no, which meals lack protein and fat?

   _____

   What can you do to add protein and fat to your meals and snacks?

   _____

   _____

   _____

3. Did you consume more than three servings of carbohydrate-containing foods at a meal or snack? Check the PCOS Food Exchange List if needed.

   If no, limiting carbohydrates, especially refined ones, will help you improve your insulin levels.

   If yes, at what meals do you exceed three servings of carbohydrate-containing foods?

   _____

   _____

   What can you do to make your meals and snacks more balanced?

   _____

   _____

   _____

4. Did you have more than two servings of refined carbohydrates per day?

   If no, you are working at improving your insulin resistance.

   If yes, do you notice a pattern of when you consume the refined foods?

   _____

   _____

   _____

   _____

   Did anything trigger you to eat these foods?

   _____

   _____

   _____

What can you do in the future to reduce your intake of these foods?

_____

_____

_____

_____

5. Did you have at least two servings of fruit each day and three servings of vegetables?

    If yes, keep it up! Eating at least five fruits and vegetables each day can improve insulin resistance, lower your blood pressure and cholesterol levels as well as improve your overall health.

    If no, what gets in the way of you eating fruits and vegetables?

_____

_____

_____

_____

What can you do to increase your consumption of fruits and vegetables?

_____

_____

_____

_____

6. During the three-day period did you eat any fatty fish (i.e., salmon, halibut, trout) or did you take a flaxseed or fish oil supplement of at least 1 gram each day?

_____

_____

If yes, you are eating a diet rich in omega-3 fatty acids, which can improve insulin resistance and lower triglyceride and cholesterol levels.

If no, what ways can you increase your consumption of omega-3 fatty acids? Would you benefit from taking a fish oil supplement?

_____

_____

_____

_____

7. How many glasses of water did you drink each day? _____

Did you consume any sweetened beverages (i.e., regular soda or juice)?

_____

If no, you are doing a good job avoiding simple sugars in sweetened beverages.

If yes, consuming sweetened beverages will spike your insulin levels quickly. What can you do to decrease your intake of sweetened beverages?

_____

_____

_____

_____

8. Examine the numbers you circled for your levels of hunger and satisfaction. Did you eat past the point of fullness or binge eat?

_____

If yes, when did the incidents occur and how?

_____

_____

_____

_____

Can you name strategies to help you manage eating past fullness or bingeing?

_____

_____

_____

_____

Did you wait until you were starving to eat? _____

If yes, when did the incidents occur and how?

_____

_____

_____

_____

Take a look at where you ate your food. Where you sitting in front of a TV or computer screen, or did you eat while you were driving?

_____

If you answered yes to these questions, you may have difficulty eating mindfully. If you are distracted during meals or engage in emotional eating, you may find it hard to stop when you feel satisfied. We will discuss these topics more in Chapter 7.

9. Did you notice any beliefs, thoughts or judgments that affected your eating? For example: "I shouldn't have eaten that." "I'm so fat!" "I already ate one cookie, might as well have another." List them here:

_____

_____

_____

_____

How can you challenge these thoughts, beliefs and judgments?

_____

_____

_____

_____

10. What else did you observe about your eating patterns and intake?

_____

_____

_____

_____

11. Keeping daily food journals is an effective way to monitor your eating and manage weight. Would you be willing to continue keeping a food journal each day? Why or why not?

_____

_____

_____

_____

12. During the past three days, were you physically active more than once?

_____

_____

_____

If yes, keep up the good work! Regular physical activity is a very effective way to improve your insulin levels.

If you weren't physically active more than once, why?

_____

_____

_____

_____

COMMITTING TO CHANGE

Chances are you didn't buy this book unless you were serious about making changes in your life. This book is a workbook. It provides information but also requires work on your own part. You have been given information on what PCOS is, why you need to make changes and how you can do it. You even gave yourself ideas on what you could do. Now it's time to put these ideas into practice.

Write down five goals (related to eating and/or exercise) that you can commit to today. Goals should be attainable and realistic. For example, if you are not a runner, committing to running three miles everyday is not realistic. Make your goals measurable, meaning assign a numeric value to them. For example, I will eat three pieces of fruit each day or eat breakfast five mornings this week or walk 10 minutes each day after work.

Goal 1.

I will

_____

_____

_____

Goal 2.

I will

_____

_____

_____

Goal 3.

I will

_____

_____

_____

Goal 4.

I will

_____

_____

_____

Goal 5.

I will

_____

_____

_____

After you meet the goals, set more goals that are attainable, realistic and measurable.

WORKING WITH A REGISTERED DIETITIAN

Working with a dietitian can offer guidance on food and diet recommendations for your specific needs. A dietitian can also assess your eating habits and give you objective and reliable nutrition information. Dietitians can help you improve your eating and help you become a more mindful eater. Women with PCOS have unique nutritional concerns requiring specialized information. To find a dietitian in your area, visit The American Dietetic Association website at www.eatright.org. When scheduling your appointment, make sure your dietitian specializes in treating PCOS.

CHAPTER 5

PCOS AND STRESS....
WHAT'S THE DEAL???

STRESS? Stress? Stress? What does stress have to do with Polycystic Ovary Syndrome? Stress has a great impact on how you experience PCOS. Stress levels affect mood, and how the hormonal and immune systems function. Stress can also influence how and where you gain weight, as well as your fertility. Are you struggling with mood instability, weight gain, hormonal functioning or infertility problems? This chapter discusses the relationship between stress and PCOS, and most importantly, what you can do to change your life.

BELIEFS ABOUT STRESS

If I gathered everyone who was reading this book into one room at the same time, and asked the question, "What stresses you out?" how many different answers do you think we'd have? We might have some commonalities such as work, body or relationships, but specifically, we'd probably have as many answers as we do people. Stress is an interesting concept because it means something different to everyone.

Often, when you think of stress, you think of events or situations that are negative or unpleasant. Negative stressors are things in your environment you might want to avoid or wish would never happen. Some examples of unpleasant or negative stressors might be running late for an important appointment or having an argument with a loved one. However, stress can also occur when anticipating or experiencing positive events. Positive stressors, such as purchasing your first home, having a baby or going on vacation are all wonderful events, and yet can create chaos and turmoil in your life.

Do you believe that only major events are "stress worthy"? Do you have judgments about the type of events that cause you stress? Do you have the thought that buying a car is a stress worthy event, but not buying sunglasses or socks? What other thoughts do you have about what is or is not stressful? What creates stress for you? Is it missing a deadline or being unemployed? Could it be getting a promotion, a first date, or maybe thinking about having a child? Think about what causes you stress and write them down here:

_____   _____

_____   _____

_____   _____

_____   _____

_____   _____

Did listing those stressors leave you pretty stressed out? If it did, where did you feel the stress? Did you feel your heart race or your palms sweat? Did your face get hot? Did you notice a swarm of judgments and negative thoughts fill your head? If you did, you're probably exhausted just thinking of them. If not, what did you notice? Take a minute to think about that. Did the list come easily? Did you struggle? Write down what you noticed here:

_____

_____

_____

_____

Stressors come in all sizes, shapes and colors. For some, stress is prompted by a physical event or change in environment such as a physical trauma, not having a nutritionally balanced diet, a nasty headache, poor air quality or an outdated eyeglass prescription. For others, stress can be prompted by the belief that things should be different then how they are. This stress can often be experienced as a tension or state of confusion. This confusion might be because there is a discrepancy between your thoughts about your life and where you actually might be in your life. Do you think you have been grateful enough to your parents or that you should be better at your job? Are you single and believe you should be married already?

WHAT HAPPENS WHEN I'M STRESSED OUT?

Stress is a concept that's been talked about for generations. As early as 1940, the term "distress" was used to describe those things in our life that cause tension and negative stress. The concept of stress can be described in one of two ways: theoretically and physiologically. This chapter reviews both so that you can get a clearer picture of what occurs when you experience stress.

Theoretically, your mind and body go through a transformation when it is met with a stressful event. Your body needs to somehow adapt to this new information and accommodate it. General Adaptation Syndrome (GAS) explains how you might confront stress, adapt to it and then move on (Figure 5.1).

Theoretically, your first response to a stressor is **"alarm."** This is when your body prepares itself for "fight or flight." This automatic response from the sympathetic nervous system activates whenever your body is faced with danger. You might recognize the fight or flight response if you think about a time when your heart raced or your eyes opened wider (pupil dilation) after hearing something stressful. Alarm occurs as the first response to a stressor.

Your body then enters into the **"stage of resistance."** In this stage, you are playing a "tug of war" with the stressful information. The information, or intense condition of alarm, is too much to tolerate all at once, so as a protective measure, your mind and body are slowly acclimating to the situation. This process of accepting and resisting is critical for the adaptation of stressful information because without the slow digestion of information, we would not be able to function.

Lastly, if the stressor persists, you will experience **"exhaustion."** Fatigue and weakness are hallmarks of this stage, and exist because the process of adapting to a stressor has truly depleted you.

Figure 5.1. General Adaptation Syndrome.

GENERAL ADAPTATION SYNDROME

- **Alarm reaction** – The response to the introduction of a stressor
- **Stage of resistance** – The process of adapting to a stressor
- **Exhaustion** – The aftereffects of stress is often fatigue and weakness

HPA system- stress on a physical level

While GAS describes what happens to you on a theoretical level, there is also a neurological and chemical process occurring. The physiological process of adapting to stress is mediated by the hypothalamus-pituitary-adrenal system (HPA). The HPA system governs the amount and kind of response the body produces to combat stress.

When you encounter stress, you produce cortisol, glucose, hormones and other chemicals to give your body that little extra "something" to get you through the experience. The increase in cortisol (the stress hormone) stimulates gastric acid activity, acts like a diuretic (which is why you might make more trips to the bathroom), increases blood pressure and aids short-term memory. Cortisol regulates how much energy we have by gathering carbohydrates, fats or proteins in the body and then sends the energy to where the body needs it most. The added increase in glucose gives extra energy to sustain any physiological demands the stress might require.

When stressful situations linger, or when you might not be managing the emotions/beliefs that result from the stress, the HPA system begins to work overtime. It's as if the switch that turned on the HPA system gets stuck in the "ON" position and the motor continually runs. This prolonged exposure to stress creates numerous physiological and emotional problems. The human body is then more vulnerable to germs, viruses and infections. Excessive exposure to cortisol can lead to heart disease, disrupted metabolism, impaired digestion, memory impairment and the destruction of healthy muscle and bone.

Specifically, the HPA system works like this (see Figure 5.2): You encounter a stressor. This stressor could be an interpersonal situation, something that occurred in the environment or something that happens intrapersonally (that is, within yourself like a memory or a thought). You may have thoughts about this stressor that include beliefs and appraisals. This process of thinking about the event stimulates the hypothalamus, the gland that bridges the brain and the endocrine system. Once stimulated, the hypothalamus excretes corticotrophin-releasing hormone (CRH). CRH stimulates the pituitary gland, which is a hormone producing gland embedded in the bones at the base of the skull. When the pituitary gland gets stimulated, it releases adrenocorticotrophic hormone (ACTH) into the bloodstream. With the release of ACTH into the blood, the adrenal glands (located above the kidneys) create and release corticoids. These corticoids, or stress hormones, come in two forms, and the one that we are interested in is called glucocorticoids. Glucocortocoids have the ability to both reduce and suppress immune system functioning and also stimulate glucose into the body. Glucocorticoids can also lead to infertility issues if the HPA system lingers by stimulating or suppressing the sex/growth hormones.

Figure 5.2. How your body responds to stress.

WHAT'S IT MEAN TO BE "STRESSED OUT"?

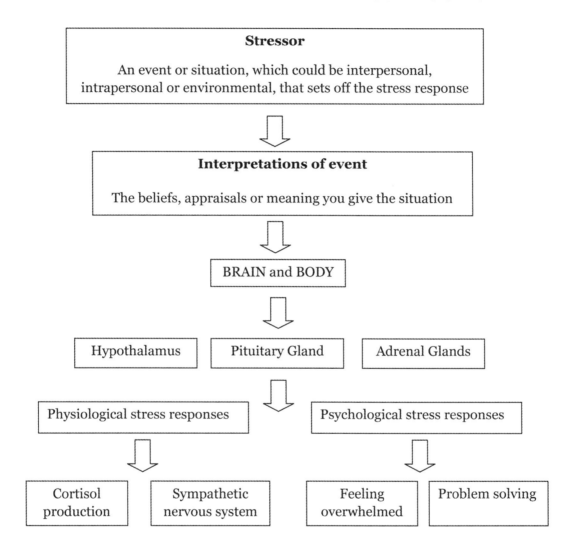

Prolonged stress leads to:

Physiological
- Disturbed immune system
- Cardiac problems
- High blood pressure
- Weight gain/weight loss
- Serotonin depression

Psychological
- Depression and anxiety
- Irritability, frustration, anger
- Confusion and memory loss
- Fatigue, anhedonia, apathy
- PTSD or problematic coping

Good old cortisol

Cortisol, which has been nicknamed the "stress hormone," plays a large role in what you might experience as a stress response. Cortisol is released by the adrenal gland during the normal stress response and is a necessary element in our lives. High cortisol levels interfere with progesterone, which is essential because progesterone is one of the precursors to the steroid hormones including estrogen and testosterone. Cortisol is also crucial for proper uterine and breast development. The problem is that cortisol and progesterone compete for the same cell receptors and when this occurs for too long, problems with menstruation and estrogen imbalance can develop, which may contribute to infertility.

Cortisol is not the bad guy. While there is some controversy among researchers about the role of cortisol metabolism in women with PCOS, cortisol levels are not typically elevated in women except when there is a significant stress reaction.

How stress affects women with PCOS

You have learned how stress impacts a human body. Since many women with PCOS struggle with insulin, glucose, infertility, sex/growth hormones and food, it is only fitting to discuss how stress might affect women with PCOS. Studies have shown that women with high cortisol levels consume more calories than women with low levels. In other words, when stress is high, you eat more. In fact, you may even eat more sweet sugary foods when cortisol is high. When cortisol levels are too high for too long, insulin resistance can result. This is because the insulin can't effectively complete the job of transporting glucose into the cells.

Women who have difficulty eating a "daily balanced diet" might be the first to increase their food consumption under stress. Studies have shown that women who restrict their food calories on a regular basis tend to increase their food consumption under stress as well. This is especially important since food manipulation and calorie restriction is a commonly used behavior in women with PCOS. These findings suggest that the "stress-eat" reaction is likely to last longer in women with PCOS who have been utilizing food restriction as a coping strategy or weight gain stabilizer.

Studies have also shown that mood is greatly affected by food consumption. There is actually an increase in how frequently you experience negative moods after stress-related food consumption. This cycle can feel like a Catch-22. Cortisol levels might be increasing your stress, which might be increasing your urge to eat to relieve the stress, only to leave you feeling bad after you eat.

Think back. Do you reach for sweet foods when you feel stressed? Do you have judgments about your tendency to do this? Did you think this pattern of stress-response food consumption was a reflection about your character or will power? If you did blame yourself for this behavior, you're not alone.

TIPS FOR THE STRESSFUL LIFE

Now that you know why stress is important and how your body reacts to stress, what can you do about it? Since you can't live a stress-free life, you need strategies to cope. The goal in stress reduction is to influence the process by which the stress reaction occurs (see Figure 5.2). There are many was to intervene in this process. Interventions could be placed at the beginning of the process or at the physiological level. As you read through the many strategies presented, think about what might be effective for you.

If you begin the intervention process when a stressor is first presented, you might be interfering here (see Figure 5.3):

Figure 5.3. What is a stressor?

Stressor
An event or situation, which could be interpersonal, intrapersonal or environmental, that sets off the stress response

If you are unaware of the prompting event for your stress, you may find yourself spending a considerable amount of time ruminating, or thinking a lot about your experience. It is human nature to make sense out of why thoughts, feelings or behaviors are present. Once the source of the stress is identified, the intensity of the stress response might decrease. Knowing why the stress response began equips you to use additional coping strategies for the stressor. The more information the better!

Restructure values and demands

Stress is often caused by demands placed upon you or in the way your values play out in your life. Demands are expectations placed on you by others because they believe that they are important. A demand might be having family members insist you attend a family party or being told to complete a particular piece of work in half the time you expected. A value is something that YOU think is important. A value might be eating whole grains instead of processed white flour, or it might be speaking your mind when you believe an injustice has occurred. Incorporating some of your values into your daily life is important. Restructuring and re-prioritizing demands and values can reduce the amount of pressure you feel. A "less is more" philosophy could help reduce the amount of stressful events in your life. Less is more might mean reducing your demand load and increasing your priorities and values. Take a minute to write down some ways you could do this:

_____

_____

_____

Stressors that are identified and structured are much easier to manage then those that are unknown and overwhelming. The next place of intervention involves the thoughts and meaning that you give to the stressor (see Figure 5.4).

Figure 5.4. Stessor-interpretaton relationship.

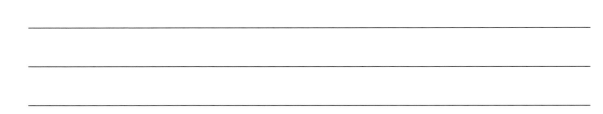

Our brains are designed to be thought churning machines, and as such your brain is no different. Your brain is constantly having thoughts about what happens, and why it happens or focused highly on some things and not enough on others. Here are some strategies to help with your interpretations of stressful events:

Question interpretations and myths

The way you interpret situations, or the way in which you assess or appraise your experience, affects how you feel. When you are aware of your expectations, the "shoulds", "the have to's" and "the musts," you can challenge your beliefs about them and reduce your stress. What are some of your "should's, have to's, or must's" do? List them:

_____

_____

_____

Use Humor

Laughter really is the best medicine. All of us get so engrossed in our world that we tend to forget the bigger picture. Life is more than the problems you have. Try to bring humor into your life and don't take yourself and your situation so seriously. What are some ways you could find humor in your current situation and with whom could you do this?

_____

_____

_____

_____

Self-validation and compassion exercises

You might think that being hard on yourself during times of stress will motivate you to work hard, but it will actually increase your anxiety and depression as well as decrease your long-term motivation. Having compassion for yourself, while difficult, reduces your negative critical thoughts and decreases shame and guilt. Recognizing that you are doing the best you can helps to problem solve more effectively. What self-validating messages could you give yourself today? In what situations would you benefit from hearing them? Write them down here:

Self-validating messages:

_____

_____

_____

_____

Times when I could benefit from hearing them:

_____

_____

_____

_____

Smelling the Roses

Go to the movies. Smell some flowers. Get your nails done. Take a mental health day from work. Play at the park. A day filled with enjoyable activities can be a more enjoyable day. Include an enjoyable activity in your schedule every day and give yourself permission to enjoy it.

Five things I really enjoy doing:

1. _____

2. _____

3. _____

4. _____

5. _____

Talk about your thoughts and feelings

Having a safe place to go to or talking with supportive people when you are feeling stressed out really helps. We all need a "shoulder to lean on and an ear to bend" from time to time. Talking about your stress helps you process the experience in a new and sometimes beneficial way. Be mindful of how frequently you refrain from sharing your experience and whether or not it contributes to your stress.

People I could feel supported by are:

_____

_____

_____

_____

Journaling

If you can't connect with someone when you need support the most or if you think others won't understand what you're going though, try journaling. Journaling can often give you a forum to express yourself in a safe and private environment. Keeping a journal or a log of your thoughts and experiences helps sort out the prompting events and interpretations as well as the feelings and aftereffects. You can write it and toss it or re-read it from time to time to see how things have changed or stayed the same.

If you've tried the strategies aimed at influencing the stressors in your life and you continue to feel the effects of stress like poor concentration, loss of sleep or racing thoughts, then you read on. The next level of intervention influences the stress process at the brain/body level (see Figure 5.5).

Figure 5.5. Stressor-interpretation-body relationship.

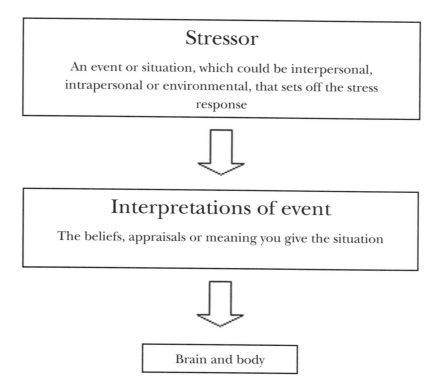

Mindfulness practices or relaxation techniques

Mindfulness-meditation practice and relaxation techniques help reduce stress by interrupting the sympathetic nervous system (see Figure 5.2). These exercises slow down breathing, help to regulate your heart rate and influence the amount of oxygen that circulates through your body. Additionally, these techniques slow down and regulate the centers in your brain responsible for attention and executive functioning which in turn influences the release of the chemicals and hormones.

The following are a few examples of some mindfulness activities that you can do. To prepare for these activities, find a place where you can sit uninterrupted for a short period of time. Sit in a comfortable position. Eyes can be open or closed. If open, find a place in the room where you can fix your gaze comfortably.

- Listen to the sounds in your environment and concentrate on them. Notice not just the sounds, but also the spaces between the sounds. Listen to them fade in and out. Do this for 5 minutes.
- Imagine yourself in a park near a stream or at the ocean. Notice the breeze, the trees and the environment. Breathe deeply as you take in the sights, smells and sounds.
- As you breathe, count your inhalations. Go from 1 to 10. When you get to 10, count backward to one. Repeat. Do this with your eyes closed for approximately 5 minutes. When you notice yourself beyond 10, smile, acknowledge that you lost count, and start again with one.
- Think about your favorite beverage. Mindfully prepare it. Notice the smells, temperatures, the sounds and the experience of anticipation. Focus all your attention on this daily process. Notice when your attention drifts to other things and gently bring it back to your imaginary drink.
- Repeat a self-validating message to yourself as you inhale. Be mindful of thoughts, feelings and sensations as you do this. Be sure to come back to the self-validating message. Notice judgments or beliefs that may interfere with being believing it.
- Imagine yourself handling your stress effectively. How would you like to be handling this stress? What interferes with that? Take a few minutes to think about what you would need to handle the situation effectively. Would you need support, time, resources, sleep, money? How could you problem solve those things?

_____

_____

_____

_____

- Do progressive muscle relaxation (PMR) exercises. Teach your muscles how to relax. Pay attention to each of the following muscle groups one at a time. Then deliberately apply tension to each area by flexing the muscle, then you release the tension and notice how the muscle relaxes. As always, check with your physician before doing PMR to determine if you have any physical ailments that might become more problematic or exacerbated by the practice.

    - Feet and legs (right then left)
    - Hands (right then left)
    - Forearms (right then left)
    - Stomach
    - Chest

- Neck and shoulders
- Face (mouth, forehead, eyes)

Other mindfulness practices or relaxation techniques that you know and love:

_____

_____

_____

Biofeedback

Biofeedback is the process of making physical changes to your body based on information or signals. First, information is acquired through an apparatus or machine about a particular physical function. A blood pressure machine gives information about the rate of blood flow in and out of the heart. A pulse oximeter gives information about oxygen levels in the blood. Both of these, the rate of blood flow and the oxygen levels in your blood can be influenced by your behavior. By breathing slowly and deeply, you can lower your heart rate and increase oxygen flow. Biofeedback is readily available in video game form and is terrific for reducing your physiological stress response, treating headaches, lowering blood pressure, treating irritable bowel syndrome and more. Biofeedback resources are probably available in your area. Ask your medical doctor or psychologist for more information.

Balanced Diet

Eating a balanced nutritionally sound diet protects against many negative influences. A well nourished body is more resilient then a vitamin deprived body. We're not suggesting you should eliminate all chocolate or caffeine, but moderation is the key. See Chapters 1 through 4 for some more tips about balancing your diet.

Exercise

Exercise has anti-depressant effects. It is good for strengthening the body and the mind. It activates our bodies and our brains by distributing oxygen, glucose and neuro-chemicals to the areas that need it. Exercise releases accumulated toxins in the body, helps you sleep better and releases endorphins that help you overcome some of your stressful events. The key to exercise as a stress management technique is to have fun, and to do it in moderation. You should only do what your body is capable of doing, not what your brain thinks you "should" do. Remember, exercise needs to be an effective strategy, not another source of stress. As always, check with your physician before doing any new exercise, especially if you have any physical ailments or muscular issues that might become more problematic or exacerbated by the practice.

Fun exercise/activities are:

_____

_____

_____

Massage Therapy

Massage therapy loosens up the muscles and releases toxins stored in them. Through massage, we experience physical relaxation and experience internal quiet time. Resources for this are:

_____

_____

_____

Acupuncture

While originating in Chinese medicine, Acupuncture is growing in popularity in the West. According to the principles of Chinese medicine, stress interrupts or blocks the flow of energy throughout the body. The "back up" causes tension and pain. Acupuncture helps by releasing the block, allowing the energy to flow smoothly, therefore eliminating the pain and tension.

Hopefully this chapter helped you feel a little less stressed and more equipped to handle the stressors in your life. Can you commit to doing something about your stress now? Can you commit to doing something different this week? If so, then you're off to a great start. Take a minute and list five things you are willing to do THIS WEEK!

1. _____

2. _____

3. _____

4. _____

5. _____

CHAPTER 6

BODY IMAGE AND PCOS

"If only I looked different. I wish I looked like the women I see at work. They don't ever have to worry about a thing. They can wear or eat whatever they want. I am so ugly."

"My body is my enemy. No matter what I do, it doesn't matter. My belly is big even though I barely eat. I grow hair where I'm not supposed to, and the pimples just show up unannounced. I hate the way I look."

"Nobody understands what it's like. I'm always afraid that people are looking at me... judging my body...thinking I'm grotesque. I see the way they look at me. I look at myself that way, why wouldn't they."

DOES this sound familiar? Many women with PCOS feel the same way about their bodies. Negative body image is a frequent issue in women with PCOS and can greatly interfere with your self-care, your self-esteem and even your relationships. If you struggle with negative thoughts about your body, then this chapter is going to be very important for you. By the end of this chapter you will:

- Understand what "body image" means,
- Identify how negative body image impacts your life,
- Learn how to challenge the thoughts and beliefs you have about your body,
- Learn how to appreciate the body you have.

WHAT IS BODY IMAGE?

Body image is the way you perceive your body. This may be different than how your body actually looks or how your body actually functions. Often times, your perception of your body is completely opposite of reality. For example, when you read the three quotes at the beginning of this chapter, you may have assumed certain characteristics about that person. You may have assumed she had excessive hair or belly fat because this is what she's complaining about. However, it is possible that the woman is average sized. She may be free of unwanted hair. She may look like anyone else. What did you think she looked like?

People often assume that the way they feel about their bodies is the way they actually look. But feelings may not be an accurate reflection of reality. Emotions are not lie detector tests. Instead, they are experiences and perceptions that are based on the way you interpret information.

The truth is there are no "perfect" bodies and no perfect body feature. Intellectually you might know this, but emotionally it might be another story. You might have mixed ideas about your body as well. The mix up often begins when you create myths, or stories about what is and what isn't and then place pressure on yourself to live up to these expectations. You might feel judged or inferior because you haven't lived up to the expectations you created. It is possible that you've created a body image myth and that you have certain beliefs about your size or shape that deviate from the "expectations".

Judgments, beliefs, interpretations, perceptions and thoughts are all words to describe your body image myth. They are ideas put together by your brain to make sense or to understand why something is the way it is. For example, someone could tell you that you have PCOS because you were born in a month beginning with the letter "J". Hopefully, not many of you would believe that because as of today we don't have any research to substantiate that "J" months predict PCOS. If you did believe this, consider the impact of thinking or believing this thought, and what might be the consequence of thinking that way. The same is true for our body image myths. You hold a pattern of thought or a particular way in which you think that contributes to the myth. This way of thinking or "cognitive pattern" can be very disruptive and sometimes distorted.

NEGATIVE BODY IMAGE AND THE BODY IMAGE MYTH

Negative body image could have an effect on the way you live. This image could interfere with your willingness to take your medication because of the expectations or judgments you have about taking it. This same negative body image could get in the way of following some dietary guidelines because of judgments you might have about hunger. It can also influence your social life. If you refrain from going out with friends or avoid the companionship of an intimate other because you're having a "fat" day or refuse to exercise because you're ashamed to leave the house, then negative body image is an issue. Negative body image impacts us all in different ways. When you have PCOS, and need to be pro-active in the care of your body, caring for your negative body image is even more critical.

Figure 6.1. Body Image Myths.

Body Image Myths

Read the following statements. Place a mark on the line if you have these thoughts.

_____ 1.   There is a perfect body type.

_____ 2.   All of the thoughts, feelings and judgments I have about my body are true.

_____ 3.   If I could just stop eating then my life would be better.

_____ 4.   I shouldn't go out socially looking the way I do.

_____ 5.   My life would be happier and more complete if I was thinner.

_____ 6.   If I look this way then I must have done something to cause it.

_____ 7.   My body is my enemy.

_____ 8.   It's hopeless. I can't make any changes to my body.

_____ 9.   Other (write in your own):_____

How many myths did you check off? _____

Are you willing to examine each belief you endorsed? If you're still reading, CONGRATULATIONS! Your curiosity about your beliefs is the first step in changing them.

Now that you know which beliefs are affecting the way you view your body, let's take a closer look at them and try to understand where they came from, what maintains them, and what you can do about it. Start by writing down the first body image myth (BIM) you checked off here:

_____

BIRTH OF THE BODY IMAGE MYTH

Do you wonder when you began to feel badly about your body? Write down the first memory that involved the BIM you wrote above. Be sure to identify where you were, who was there and what was said.

_____

_____

_____

_____

_____

_____

_____

During your life, you "learn" about the world and yourself through your experiences. You encounter things that make you feel good and things that make you feel bad. Through this process, you learn to seek more of what you like, and less of what you don't. As an adult, you have control over many of these choices. You can choose your friends, activities, work, clothing and food. As a child though, you had much less control over the environments and situations in which you were placed. Often, the seeds of negative BIM take root during that childhood inter- and intrapersonal learning.

Culturally, society teaches children that appearance is critical. In the United States, for example, we have certain norms for appropriate dress and weight. Even if parents don't embrace the standard norms, children are bombarded with these messages from the moment they are born.

I'll never forget the time my then 3-year-old daughter dressed herself in a fancy dress, snow boots and a baseball cap. Then we went shopping. I was amazed at the number grimaces I received from disapproving passers-by. That moment was a clear indication of just how "hung up" society (American society) is about appearance. Even though my daughter and I were happy about her choice in clothing, many people who walked by her were openly offended. For them, my daughter's clothing was "wrong". Take a minute and think about the birth of your myth. Was it influenced by the social and cultural norms of your childhood? Was there a belief about what was wrong or right or about how you should look or shouldn't look? Take a moment and write down your thoughts here:

_____

_____

_____

_____

_____

_____

_____

_____

Puberty is another time that negative BIM's emerge. In adolescence, our bodies are changing and growing. Add raging hormones and our bodies begin changing drastically. Girls develop breasts and hips. They start to menstruate and get acne. As the size, shape and function of our body changes, you may have had thoughts and feelings about the rate that these changes occur. For many girls, those thoughts and fears could have been about being "different" then everyone else. During that time, many young girls just want to fit in, or be similar to everyone, and ostracized by no one. Everyone wants to be accepted, included, thought about and wanted. Did you feel different? What was this time like for you? Take a minute and think about the birth of your myth, was it born here? Write down your thoughts about it:

_____

_____

_____

_____

_____

_____

For many, getting the PCOS diagnosis comes at the end of a long journey. A journey filled with well meaning doctors who offered advice such as "just loose a few pounds" or "exercise more" when you asked about your weight. Or maybe you were not taken seriously when you discussed your irregular periods and were advised to just take the pill. And maybe cosmetic surgery was offered when you brought up the unexplained hair growth.

For many, the journey to reach a diagnosis exacerbated an underlying depression and may have triggered overall body dissatisfaction. What was your journey like? Take a minute and think about your BIM. Was it born here? Write down a few thoughts:

_____

_____

_____

_____

_____

_____

_____

Myths have so many origins. Understanding where the myths emerged is valuable. Understanding how the myths came to be gives you insight into them and hopefully some compassion for yourself. This compassion may help you understand that your beliefs developed out of real experiences, real thoughts and perhaps real fears. Without exploration, these myths have "sticking power." When we identify, explore and challenge the myths, we break the bond that has kept them stuck for so long.

CHALLENGING THE BODY IMAGE MYTHS

Choose a myth from Figure 6.1 that you are willing to explore and challenge. Answer the following questions about your negative BIM. Feel free to add another sheet of paper if needed.

The myth I am exploring and challenging is:

_____

1. **Environment.** For many people their beliefs about their body become more frequent and prevalent in the company of certain people, stressors or during particular events. Does this happen to you? Are there times when you might have particular beliefs and times when you do not? Do emotions, thoughts or people influence this myth?

_____

_____

_____

_____

_____

Being mindful of the connection between the environment and your myth is the first way to change the relationship. There might be particular stressors or people that prompt your BIM. If you follow the suggestions in Chapter 5 for dealing with stressors in your life, you'll be on your way to changing the impact of the environment.

2. **Truth.** Is it possible that your belief is not "completely" true? Often myths are fear based or based on another emotion so they are not 100% realistic? Do you notice yourself having the thought: "If I think it, it must be true."?

_____

_____

_____

_____

Being able to notice when the myth is not true is the first step to knowing that your belief is not "the way it is." Perhaps you are focusing more time and energy on noticing when the myth does occur than when it does not. Remembering times when it hasn't been true will help you challenge this myth.

3. **All or nothing thinking**. Problematic thinking can often be black and white, all or nothing, or very extreme. Is your myth one of those thoughts? Examples of all or nothing thinking include thinking that something is always a problem, that it will never change or that things are hopeless?

_____

_____

_____

_____

4. **Rules.** Is your BIM part of a set of rules you created? Do you have rules about the way things "should be?" Do these rules apply to everyone or just you? Are these rules too strict for your life right now? Are there ways of changing the rules so that they are less rigid, more flexible and more encompassing of the whole picture?

_____

_____

_____

_____

When changing rules that interfere and influence your body image it is important to realize that you created them. You created them and you have the power to change them. These rules may have served you at one point in your life, but perhaps they are hindering your life now. Consider this as a possibility.

5. **Mindful perspective.** Is there information that you "forget" or neglect to consider important when you think about your body image myth? Do you "leave out" information, like considering the impact that untreated PCOS might have on your body or your current hormonal levels? Is there information that you might need in order to get a more realistic idea of how it all fits together?

_____

_____

_____

_____

Being mindful of all the facts before making judgments about your body is critical. Information gathering is important because it can provide room for you to have compassion for your current situation and body shape, size or type.

6. **Selective attention.** Think about your life at the current moment. Do you have a career, intimate relationship, other relationships, hobbies or passions? Are you giving these aspects of your life as much attention as you do your body? Is there a disproportionate ratio of time scrutinizing and magnifying the importance of this myth?

_____

_____

_____

_____

When you think about the amount of time you dedicate to thinking about your body image myth vs. the amount of time you think about other aspects of your life, it should be disproportionate. That is, your LIFE should get the majority of attention. Make the choice to "interrupt" your attention to negative body image with activities that you enjoy.

7. **Minimizing.** To believe this myth, is there information that you discount or minimize? Have you been told by others that your myth isn't true? Do you find that when people say it's not true that you don't believe it or think it "doesn't count"?

    _____

    _____

    _____

    _____

    Minimizing information is like not seeing the "big picture." Ask yourself the question: "What are the facts of the situation?" Once you know all the facts then it will be easier to discern which information is relevant in making body image choices.

8. **Self-blame.** Do you often think that this myth is your "fault"? Do you believe you deserve or have caused your body or diagnosis? Do you blame yourself for the way your body is now? Does it motivate you toward action or does it keep you paralyzed in the cycle of self-blame and shame? What would be more effective?

    _____

    _____

    _____

    _____

    _____

    Blaming yourself for your illness will not help. Being harsh or judgmental about the way your body looks or functions will only keep you paralyzed. Instead, choose a position of compassion and warmth. Have compassion for how hard you are working at making a difference in your life and your body.

The myth re-visited

What did you notice about your BIM as you went through the process of answering those questions? Did it become less "absolute" and maybe a bit more flexible? Could you re-write the myth in a way that is more accepting of you as a whole person?

_____

_____

_____

_____

_____

Now that you've completed the exercise for one of your BIM, perform the exercise for the remaining myths you checked off.

APPRECIATING THE BODY I HAVE?

Negative body image is learned. We learn it from a variety of sources, and every culture teaches it differently. For example, negative body image in Caucasian American women is not the same as in African American women. In the process of learning how to appreciate the body you have, it is important to recognize the impact not appreciating it has on you. Research tells us that women with PCOS report more depression and more body dissatisfaction then women without it. Body dissatisfaction might contribute to the depression! Negative pervasive thoughts and feelings about our bodies can lead to depression, disappointment and anxiety. Is this the case for you?

If you want to move away from depression and anxiety about your body you must embrace the idea that your body isn't "ALL BAD." In fact, there are many amazing things your body is doing right now. Be thankful that your heart beats or you fight off infection. Consider the following things your body does for you every day:

- Fights infection
- Moves you forward or to the top of a hill
- Stays awake so you could drive home safely
- Learns new skills
- Heals bruises
- Sticks by you during your entire existence
- Gives you a new sensual sensation
- Converts matter into usable energy through metabolism
- Gets stronger

- Keeps working despite pain
- Expresses a strong emotion through your face and body language
- Makes another human being
- Soothes or comforts someone else
- Defends you from an attack or heals from an injury
- Grew into its current form from a sperm and an egg
- Releases you from pain
- Offers life in the form of blood or an organ to someone else
- Hears the sound of children laughing
- Rejuvenates during sleep
- Feels the touch of another person

Few of us are mindful of the miracles our bodies perform on a daily basis. Make a deliberate choice to shift out of a "notice everything negative" perspective to a "notice everything" perspective. Once you give yourself permission to view your body in this way, you will notice your negative BIM begin to change. Complete the exercise below to get you started with this "Notice everything about your body" philosophy.

NOTICE THE "EVERYTHING" ABOUT YOUR BODY

1. What do you like about your body? What parts feel comfortable or natural?

   _____

   _____

   _____

   _____

2. How is your body different than the "ideal" body in your mind?

   _____

   _____

   _____

   _____

3. How realistic is the "ideal" body?

_____

_____

_____

_____

_____

4. What have you done to achieve that ideal?

_____

_____

_____

_____

_____

5. What has the search for the ideal body cost you?

_____

_____

_____

_____

_____

6. What would happen if you were willing to accept your body now?

_____

_____

_____

_____

_____

7. What will you give up in life if you choose not to love your body and treat it well?

_____

_____

_____

_____

_____

This is the only body you're going to get, learn to accept it, and treat it with kindness.

CHAPTER 7

ON THE ROAD TO MINDFUL EATING

IF you're like many women with PCOS, you know you need to eat healthier and you want to, but may find yourself bingeing or emotional eating. You may even feel that changing your eating habits is hopeless because of an internal tug-of-war. For some, eating behaviors and attitudes are life-long and deeply ingrained, making them feel almost impossible to change. The reality is anyone can change their eating patterns. They just need the right motivation, support and resources. The purpose of this chapter is to do just that. First, you will learn what emotional eating is and why it's so common among women with PCOS. Then you will be offered tools to become a more mindful eater to help decrease your emotional eating. To do this, you will be encouraged to explore your connection with eating and apply ways to cope with your feelings without using food.

WHAT IS EMOTIONAL EATING?

The occasional spoonful of ice cream when we're feeling sad, blue or happy is normal. But, when it is the only way to cope with emotions, it's emotional eating. Emotional eating involves the use of food as a coping strategy for regulating intense emotions on a regular, on-going basis. This coping could be bingeing on food as a way of changing your emotion, or the opposite, restricting your eating for the same reason. If you're overwhelmed or angry and you're eating food to distract yourself from the feelings or to calm yourself, you are emotionally eating. If you avoid eating food as a way to numb yourself from feeling, you are also engaging in emotional eating. While it may feel like it helps you in the short term, using food to cope provides only a temporary fix. Answer the following questions about emotional eating.

How frequently do you...

Indicate: (N) never, (O) occasionally, (F) frequently or (C) constantly

- Binge on comfort food when you are stressed? _____

- Keep certain foods out of your house for fear of eating an entire package in one sitting? _____

- Eat to self-soothe?_____

- Eat as a distraction from life events?_____

- Use/eat food to solve interpersonal problems?_____

- Eat when you have negative thoughts about yourself or your future? _____

- Eat when you're lonely/sad/anxious? _____

- Eat after you spend time with certain people/ certain situations? _____

If you've answered frequently or constantly to at least three of these examples, then chances are that you're an emotional eater. Did you know this about yourself? If not, then what do you think now?

_____

_____

_____

PCOS AND EMOTIONAL EATING

The physiological struggle with food

Both emotional and physiological factors contribute to why women with PCOS struggle with their eating. As mentioned in the first few chapters, having high insulin causes you to have low blood sugar, which creates strong and intense cravings for carbohydrates. The cravings occur as a physiological means to raise blood sugar to normal levels. Eating refined carbohydrate foods, especially in the form of sweets, will instantly raise blood sugar. Waiting too long to eat, eating too many refined carbohydrates at once, or not having enough protein with your meals contributes to low blood sugar, giving you the urge to eat everything in sight. Your cravings may be worse before your period starts. This is mostly due to fluctuations in your sex hormone levels.

"I try not eating food all day to lose weight,
but I get so hungry that I end up bingeing."

Women with PCOS have impaired levels of ghrelin and leptin, the hormones responsible for regulating our appetite and sending out hunger and fullness cues. Having impaired levels of these hormones can cause you to eat more even when your body doesn't need more. Being mindful of your hunger and satisfaction cues will help you determine the appropriate food intake for you.

The emotional struggle with food

Using food to cope with emotions contributes to emotional eating. Often eating can be a way of zoning out, especially if your life is stress filled and you need an emotional break. Turning to food can be a temporary distraction or a time out from the current issues in your life.

Can you write examples of when:

• You turned to food in times of sadness?

_____

_____

- Food has been a source of pleasure in your life?

  _____

  _____

- You turned to sweets under stress?

  _____

  _____

- You soothed your troubles with food?

  _____

  _____

*"I hate my body. I try to be good but after a few days I only find myself
out of control with food, and it's mostly high carb stuff. I can't stop!"*

DISCONNECTED EATING

Disconnected eating occurs when you lose the physical connection that determines your food intake. This happens when you don't trust your body to regulate food intake. For instance, when you diet, you put your trust in the diet. It tells you how much to eat and what foods you can ("legal") or can't ("illegal") eat. If you have, for example, reached your number of points allowed on your plan and you're still hungry, you are supposed to ignore your hunger. If you are dieting and you crave a food that's "illegal" you can't have it. It doesn't matter if your body needs it or wants it. When you diet, you put your trust in the diet and not in yourself. This is when our eating becomes disconnected.

Diets view foods as "good" or "bad," which creates judgments about your food choices. If you have been on a very low-carbohydrate diet, you can relate to this idea. You may have read or been told that certain carbohydrate foods, including fruits and some vegetables, are bad. Yet your body relies on carbohydrates as its main energy source. Fruit and vegetables provide necessary nutrients that can reduce inflammation and lower the risk for chronic diseases. Women with PCOS may crave carbohydrates more than the average woman because of elevated insulin levels. If you crave carbohydrates and restrict them, then give in and eat them, you feel guilty. You also may feel like a failure. For some women, that "failure" can lead to bingeing on carbohydrates, an example of all-or-nothing thinking: "I already ate this brownie so I may as well finish the pan," or "It's hopeless. I'm hopeless." These are the primary reasons why some diets don't work. Diets can cause disconnection to eating and create judgments in our heads.

MINDFUL VS. MINDLESS EATING

Mindless eating, unlike emotional eating or disconnected eating, can occur without your realizing it. Mindless eating occurs when you eat without paying attention to what you are doing. It's like driving down a familiar road for the thousandth time and not remembering whether or not you stopped at all the stop signs. The trip was mindless. Your mind was elsewhere. Mindless eating is just like that. Your mind is elsewhere. This can be problematic if you are trying to pay more attention to your food choices. Answer the following questions about mindless eating.

When was the last time you...?

- Ate while working on the computer_____

- Ate while watching TV _____

- Ate while driving _____

- Ate while standing in the kitchen _____

- Ate while you were crying/yelling _____

- Walked around the house/office eating _____

- Notice you've eaten an entire bag of something without realizing it? _____

How many of them have you done this week? _____

If you answered only once, then you engaged in mindless eating. If you are engaging in this type of eating more than once each week, you may be a mindless eater.

Mindful eating is about enjoying food and nourishing your body. It's noticing the taste of food, the smell, texture, and how it feels in your body. It's about eating a variety of foods, free of judgments. Mindful eating is about being physically connected to the food you eat by recognizing and responding to your body's internal cues of hunger, satiety and fullness.

You are born with an innate mechanism to regulate your food intake. Babies do this automatically. When babies are hungry, they will cry, put fingers in their mouths, open wide or gesture for food. When a baby has had enough food to eat it will stop eating, refuse food, turn away or throw food. There's an internal physiological mechanism present at birth that sends signals to our brain indicating hunger and fullness. We all have this capability, even as adults. Hunger is your body's way of communicating that you need more energy or food. Satisfaction and fullness are signals your body coveys when it doesn't need any more energy right now.

Not trusting your body to determine how much food you need — or if you're eating is disconnected — can cause you to eat more than needed. This results in weight gain or failure to lose weight. Have you ever been watching TV or driving while you eat and suddenly the food is gone? Maybe you ate it all and didn't remember tasting it. Sometimes you don't know what it looked or smelled like. How satisfying is that? You missed out on the pleasure of several sensations. When your mind is focused on other things, your body has difficulty identifying what your body is experiencing. Your body may have needed less food but because you weren't eating mindfully, you may have eaten more than you needed. This is when problems with weight management arise.

EATING A RAISIN MINDFULLY

The following is an interesting exercise to try. You might want to begin by finding something you want to eat "mindfully". Try something small like a raisin or a cracker, or a whole food like an orange. Now, as you take this journey, be mindful of thoughts, feelings and sensations. Afterward, you can write your thoughts down if you want, but for now on just sit with your raisin and notice your thoughts as you read on. Remember, the goal is awareness, so as long as you're paying attention, you're doing it RIGHT!

Take the food (let's say it's a raisin) and place it in your hand. Just look at it for a minute. Think about how it grew, how it was packaged, transported, displayed, sold, bought, opened and now sitting in the palm of your hand. What a trip this little raisin has had. Appreciate its little life so far.

Look at it. What does it look like? Is it brown, yellow or something else entirely? Is it wrinkled or smooth? Notice its texture as the light hits it. Turn it around in your hand and really check it out. Why did you pick THIS one instead of the others? Was there something different about the way it looks?

Now take a minute and smell it. When was the last time you smelled a raisin? Does it have a smell? Have you ever smelled that before? What does it remind you of? Does it bring back any memories? Is it a brand new smell?

Slowly take the raisin and place it on your tongue. Don't CHEW IT YET!!! We still have more to go. Notice what it's like to have it just sit on your tongue. Does it roll around in your mouth? Are you salivating? Do you notice the urge to bite down on it? If you can, move it around with your tongue and notice what it feels like to be in your mouth. Notice the sound it might make as it bumps up against your teeth.

Now slowly, and I mean slowly, bite down. DON'T SWALLOW. Notice the rush of saliva that enters your mouth as the sweet juice from the raisin escapes into the cavern of your mouth. Notice the sweetness that now occupies the space. How is this contrasted to the taste you had before. Now slowly swallow. Notice the lingering taste, and urge to continue chewing. Hold off on following that urge to bite for one more second. Now chew. As your teeth macerate the flesh of the raisin, it becomes smaller and smaller. Notice this as the contents of this raisin enter your stomach and become nourishment for your body. Your body knows exactly what to do to convert that tiny raisin into fuel. Amazing!

The following questions are designed to explore your physical connection with your hunger and your ability to be a mindful eater. These questions may help you see what you need to improve. Take your time with these; maybe think about the questions during the next few days.

Exploring your relationship with food

1. What do you experience when you are hungry?

_____

_____

_____

_____

_____

2. When you're hungry, does it hit you all at once or gradually?
   Provide examples.

   _____

   _____

   _____

   _____

   _____

3. How do you know when you are comfortably full versus stuffed?
   What's the difference?

   _____

   _____

   _____

   _____

4. If you are feeling full or satisfied, can you leave food on your plate?
   Why or why not?

   _____

   _____

   _____

   _____

5. When you are hungry, how do you feel about your body?

_____

_____

_____

_____

_____

6. How do you feel about your body when you are full? If you binge eat, how do you feel after you binge?

_____

_____

_____

_____

_____

7. What happens if you are hungry and don't eat right away?

_____

_____

_____

_____

8. When was the last time you ate and were comfortably satisfied? How did that feel?

_____

_____

_____

_____

_____

9. If food did not impact your weight or your health, how would your eating style be different?

_____

_____

_____

_____

_____

10. When was the last time you ate for emotional reasons? Can you identify any events that may have triggered it?

_____

_____

_____

_____

_____

PHYSICAL CUES OF HUNGER AND FULLNESS

In Chapter 4, you were presented with food records and asked to write down your food intake for a few days, which included a hunger and satisfaction scale from 1 (completely empty) to 10 (stuffed to the max). When you did this exercise, did you notice if you had difficulty rating how hungry or full you were? If you struggle with this, the last half of this chapter will help you get more connected to your eating.

To heal the disconnection you have between your body and food, you have to be mindful of your eating. Although mindful eating sounds simple: "Eat when you're hungry and stop when you're full," it's anything but simple when you've struggled with eating and weight your whole life. The first step in being a mindful eater is practice. The raisin exercise taught you how to be more aware of food in your body. Not just the taste and texture of it, but how your body responds to it. Practicing this exercise every time you eat is one way to be more mindful of your eating.

Another way is to connect with your physiological need for food. This means recognizing how hungry you are and how satisfied you feel while you eat. These physiological needs are easily overlooked or ignored when you diet or experience intense emotions like anger or sadness. The key to mindful eating is staying in touch with internal cues of hunger and fullness. The result: Your body gets the appropriate energy it needs. Mindful eating helps better control your blood sugar and insulin levels, helping you lose weight.

The next exercise walks you through a Mindful Eating Experience, which asks you to notice your hunger and satiety signals during a meal. When you are ready, practice this exercise during meals. To start, pick one meal each day, then add more meals. Create a goal to eat mindfully most of the time.

A Mindful Eating Experience

- **Create a beautiful environment.** Use a tablecloth and attractive plates. Add flowers and unscented candles. Play music.
- **Take 1 or 2 deep cleansing breaths.** Become aware of your internal cues of hunger and appetite. Be aware of your environment, feelings, thoughts and body sensations.
- **Look at your food.** Notice the colors and textures. Be aware of your internal responses. How do you feel? Slowly bring the food up to your nose and experience its aroma.
- **Before eating, take another centered breath.**
- **Slowly take a bite.** Be aware of how the food tastes and how you feel about this food. Be aware of how the food feels in your mouth and in your body.
- **Eat slowly.** Savor the flavors. Taste the food. Chew thoroughly.
- **Breathe as you eat.** This slows down thinking and makes you aware of the sensations in your body.
- **Be aware of your satisfaction level.** Touch base with your feelings and your physical comfort level. Rate or describe how satisfied you are.

- **Stop eating at the point of maximum comfort.** Your stomach is filled, not stuffed. There is neither a sensation of hunger nor discomfort from overeating.
- **Your appetite is satisfied.** To be aware of your stopping point, eat slowly and pay attention.

EXPLORING INTERNAL CUES
OF HUNGER AND FULLNESS

We know food records may be a painful process and many people associate them with unsuccessful diets. Food records, however, can be a valuable tool to self-monitor your eating habits. In Chapter 4, you were asked to keep records and analyze your eating. Besides your food selections, the most important component of the food record is rating your degree of hunger and satisfaction. This self-monitoring tool assists you in exploring your internal cues of hunger and fullness. Not only will food records help you identify what you're feeling, it can also indicate what foods are more satisfying than others. The following are examples of food records written by women practicing mindful eating. For more detailed information about how to use food records review Chapter 4.

Cara

Cara was having difficulty being connected with her eating. Notice that she ate mindfully for breakfast: she was at Level 3, somewhat hungry, and stopped when she was satisfied at Level 7. Her breakfast satisfied her for close to four hours. At 11 a.m., she was hungry, a Level 3 on the scale, yet she didn't take the time to eat because she said she was too busy. Because she didn't eat when her body told her she needed energy, by the time she ate at 1 p.m., she reached a Level 1 - completely starving and made an unhealthy food choice. Because she was so hungry, Cara may not have taken the time to plan a healthier meal. She also ate at her desk while working and reported she didn't taste the food. Later that night when Cara was out to dinner, she felt that the meal was very satisfying and didn't overeat. She was relaxed and practiced "checking in" to rate her satisfaction level.

Cara								
Time	Food Eaten & Amount	Grains / Starches	Protein	Fats	Fruits	Vegetables	Hunger / Satisfaction	Thoughts, feelings, symptoms
6:30 AM	1 packet Plain Oatmeal 1/2 Cup Skim Milk 1 tsp sliced almonds 3/4 cup Blueberries	1	.5	1	1		1 2 ③ 4 5 6 ⑦ 8 9 10	Yummy! I like having this for breakfast
11 AM							1 2 ③ 4 5 6 7 8 9 10	Hungry but too busy to eat
1 PM	Cheesesteak and fries	4	8?	6?			① 2 3 4 5 6 7 8 ⑨ 10	Starving. Ate at my desk. Not a healthy choice. Full -- didn't taste much
6 PM	Pork, appx. 6 oz; Garden Salad w/Italian 2/3 Cup Brown Rice Steamed Vegetable 1 Glass wine	2	6	2		3	1 2 ③ 4 5 6 ⑦ 8 9 10	Out to dinner with friend. Relaxed. Mindful of how full I was getting.
Total Amount		7	14+	9+	1	3	1 2 3 4 5 6 7 8 9 10	

Becky

Becky had difficulty listening to her body. Although she was rushed, Becky said her breakfast was enough. She appeared to eat mindfully at lunch. She ate when she was at Level 3 and started getting pretty hungry. Becky also stopped eating when she was at Level 7. Again she felt rushed but enjoyed her meal. A few hours later she began eating for emotional reasons. She was overwhelmed with work and knew she wasn't hungry and ended up eating almost an entire big bag of chips. The result was her feeling very full, then guilty. This would have been a great opportunity for Becky to acknowledge feeling overwhelmed and deal with the emotion in a healthier way. Perhaps she could have taken a walk to clear her head, practiced deep breathing or talked with a co-worker.

Becky had difficulty stopping to eat at dinner. She knew she ate enough but still ate everything on her plate. Soon afterward, she ate emotionally by eating four cookies even though she was still full from dinner. She was stressed by work and felt guilty for eating everything on her plate. Becky could try alternative coping methods instead of using food.

Becky

Time	Food Eaten & Amount	Grains / Starches	Protein	Fats	Fruits	Vegetables	Hunger / Satisfaction	Thoughts, feelings, symptoms
8 AM	Banana, 2T Peanut Butter		1	2	2		1 2 ③ 4 5 ⑥ 7 8 9 10	Rushed. Felt like enough
12PM	Greek salad, 1/2 cup cottage cheese, grapes	1	2	3	1	3	1 2 ③ 4 5 6 ⑦ 8 9 10	Ate with a co-worker. Rushed but enjoyed it
2 PM	3/4 bag (big) of chips	1					1 2 3 ④ 5 ⑥ 7 ⑧ 9 10	Ate too much; overwhelmed at work. Too much to do. Wasn't hungry. Wish I hadn't eaten all that.
6:30 PM	6oz chicken and 1/2 cup pasta and olive oil, 2tsp, 1/2 cup broccoli	3	6	2		1	① 2 ③ 4 5 6 7 ⑧ 9 10	Ate too much pasta. Knew I was full but finished plate
8 PM	4 cookies	4		4			1 2 3 4 5 6 ⑦ 8 ⑨ 10	Felt like I blew it at dinner; may as well have cookies. Thinking of work
Total Amount		7	10	11	3	4		

Copyright www.PCOSnutrition.com

Sara

Sara is an example of a woman who eats mindfully. For breakfast she sat down at the table and felt satisfied with what she ate. She ate a few hours later when she was hungry and stopped again when she felt she had enough. She reported noticing how the soup was filling.

Sara ate a snack a few hours later that consisted of fruit and nuts. For dinner Sara enjoyed her meal. Although she ate everything on her plate, she wasn't stuffed. Since she craved chocolate later in the evening Sara had a reasonable serving of chocolate covered almonds. She wanted more but chose to start knitting instead.

Time	Food Eaten & Amount	Grains / Starches	Protein	Fats	Fruits	Vegetables	Hunger / Satisfaction	Thoughts, feelings, symptoms
7 AM	2 eggs 1 slice whole wheat toast 1 cup melon	1	2		1		1 2 (3) 4 5 (6)(7) 8 9 10	Satisfied Sat down to eat
11:30 AM	Grilled cheese on rye 1 cup vegetable soup	2	2	1		2	1 2 (3) 4 5 6 (7)8 9 10	At desk but shut computer monitor off Soup was filling
3 PM	Apple 8 walnuts		6	2	1		1 2 3 (4) 5 (6) 7 8 9 10	Good snack Enough
6 PM	6 oz. salmon 2/3 c. whole wheat couscous 1 cup green beans 1 tsp oil	2		1		2	1 2 (3) 4 5 6 (7)8 9 10	Enjoyed meal Ate it all
8:30 PM	8 choc covered almonds	1		2			1 2 3 (4) 5 (6) 7 8 9 10	Craved chocolate! Wanted more, but started knitting
Total Amount		6	10	6	2	4		

Sara

Copyright www.PCOSnutrition.com

A copy of the food record and hunger/satisfaction scale is located in the appendix. Make additional copies using one for each day. Have your food record available throughout the day so you remember to write down what you eat. Fill them out while eating (a great way to skillfully practice mindful eating) or soon after you've eaten while still mindful of your feelings. Don't get discouraged if you occasionally forget to write down what you ate - just move on to the next meal. Remember: no one is judging you but you. Food records are a tool to help you explore and practice eating mindfully. If you do have difficulty doing this, you may want to consider working with a registered dietitian or therapist who specializes in distorted eating.

Tips for being a more mindful eater

1. **Eat without distraction.** Turn off the TV. Move away from your computer. Don't eat in the car while driving. Consider making these rules for yourself.
2. **Check in often.** We ask others how they feel all the time, yet how often do we ask ourselves? Every so often listen to yourself and see what you need. Are you hungry or thirsty?
3. **Center yourself.** After you have sat down to eat but before you start eating, take some deep breaths to relax and calm down. Think about the food in front of you, what it looks like and how hungry you are.
4. **Slow down.** Take your time eating. If you are eating fast (to get back to something else), you won't eat mindfully. You need to taste the food, feel the texture, savor the flavor, and smell the aroma as well as you listen to internal cues of food regulation.
5. **Observe others.** Pick a couple of people you think are mindful eaters and observe them eating on several different occasions. Ask them how it feels to leave food on the plate, why they passed on a piece of birthday cake or why they finished eating something.
6. **Use food journals.** Journals may seem like an added responsibility but they keep you accountable, assess your mindful eating and show you what combinations of food satisfy you most.
7. **Practice, practice, practice!** Chances are you won't become a successful mindful eater after one or two meals. The process of discovery takes time. Don't get discouraged. Try viewing the process as an exploration of your relationship with food.

WHEN THE URGE TO EAT ISN'T ABOUT HUNGER

Each time you have an urge to eat ask yourself the following question:

Am I hungry?

If the answer is "yes", your body needs energy. You should sit down and eat slowly and mindfully. If the answer is "no", and you aren't hungry, you don't need to eat! Instead of eating, ask yourself these questions:

1. Am I mindful of any aversive feelings that I am trying to avoid? Y or N
2. Am I mindful of any thoughts that eating might distract me from? Y or N
3. Am I mindful of any recent experiences that might influence my desire to eat? Y or N
4. Am I bored? Y or N

5. Am I mindful of any other reason I might want to eat? Y or N (write it here)

_____

If you were willing to honestly answer these questions, then congratulations. Now that you know what is really going on, you have options. You can:

- Choose to distract,
- Problem solve your situation or
- Work through the emotions that trouble you.

If you feel like you can do this alone, then do so. If this is difficult to do, please contact a professional who specializes in eating disorders and emotional eating.

EMOTIONS, THOUGHTS AND EXPERIENCES

If you were looking to avoid feelings, thoughts or a recent experience, food is not the best way to do it. If you eat to numb the thoughts and feelings, you will compound the stress of the situation because after eating, you still have the original thoughts and feelings PLUS the added guilt of eating. Emotional eating might be effective in the moment, but in the long term, it causes more problems.

How does emotional eating help in the short term?

_____

_____

_____

_____

How long does it "numb out" the thoughts or feelings?

_____

_____

_____

_____

If your answer resembled anything like: "Food always takes care of my emotions" or "I find myself using food as the only way I cope," or "I don't really think about my problems because I'm always eating," then chances are it's time to talk to a professional. You might want to seek the guidance of a psychologist, psychiatrist, licensed professional counselor, social worker or a registered dietitian with a specialty in eating disorders. He or she will help you understand the role that food plays in your emotion regulation and offer new strategies and techniques to regulate your feelings.

ALTERNATIVE SELF-SOOTHING AND DISTRACTION ACTIVITIES

If you use eating and food for self-soothing or a short term distraction, there is good news: There are many activities that can take the place of eating. Many of these self-soothing and distraction techniques will get you "through the moment". Pick something on the list as a replacement to emotional or mindless eating.

- Call a friend
- Paint your nails
- Surf the internet
- Do a puzzle
- Write a letter
- Drink a cup of tea
- Listen to music
- Brush your teeth
- Garden
- Clean a closet
- Write in a journal or diary
- Take a bath
- Read a book or magazine
- Take care of someone/something
- Scrapbook
- Knit
- Paint or draw
- Go for a walk
- Look through photographs
- Light a candle
- Watch a movie
- Download new music

Can you write down three activities from the list above (or add your own suggestions) to distract you from eating?

1. _____

2. _____

3. _____

Copy these activities on another sheet of paper, hang one on your refrigerator and carry one copy with you. If those activities stop working for you, try others. The more you regularly practice these strategies, the easier you will comfort yourself without food.

Developing a healthier relationship with food doesn't happen overnight. It's an art form that gets better with practice. Performing the exercises in this chapter on a regular basis is a great way to create a new and healthier relationship with food. For more resources and books on mindful eating, please see the appendix. If you find these exercises are too challenging or difficult, seek professional treatment from a therapist and registered dietitian.

CHAPTER 8

COPING WITH INFERTILITY

ROUGHLY 7.3 million women and their partners in the United States are affected by infertility. This translates to approximately one out of every seven couples. Unfortunately, if you have PCOS, that "one" may likely be you. Infertility is the most common medical complication among women with PCOS and occurs in nearly 75% of those affected. In some cases, women are unaware of their PCOS *until they start trying* to have children. Many women who struggle to conceive may experience an enormous sense of guilt because they blame themselves. This often leaves women with an intense feeling of isolation. If you have PCOS and are struggling with infertility, you are not alone.

While PCOS is now considered a complex endocrine disorder, it was long considered a reproductive disorder. The two systems are inexorably linked. Because women with PCOS have a decreased sensitivity to insulin, which leads to the overproduction of insulin, high levels of insulin may contribute to an overproduction of androgens, which leads to irregular, infrequent menstruation and anovulation. If you aren't ovulating, you won't conceive. However, in combination with physical activity and a healthy diet, medication is available to induce ovulation and help achieve pregnancy. (See Treatment Options in this chapter).

One stressor associated with infertility is the surprise factor. When couples are ready to "start trying," few expect to encounter problems. Therefore, after a year of trying and no pregnancy to show for it (the accepted definition of infertility), feelings of dejection, confusion, frustration, hopelessness and self-blame often develop. For women with PCOS, infertility often leads them to a PCOS diagnosis, which may compound their feelings. The late diagnosis can be another source of anger, resentment or create a sense of lack of control.

Often, women with undiagnosed PCOS are told as teenagers that their irregular periods are a function of typical adolescent development. They may be prescribed an oral contraceptive to induce regular menstruation. In so doing, the pill (a mainstay of treatment for women with PCOS) unknowingly masks the symptoms that could lead to a diagnosis by decreasing androgen levels, regulating menstruation and improving hirsutism and acne. As these women are ready to conceive, they go off the pill only to re-experience irregularity and anovulation (now coupled with infertility, which they may initially blame on the many years of oral contraceptive use).

What did you feel when you first learned of your PCOS? Include the thoughts and feelings you experienced when you learned of its connection to infertility:

_____

_____

_____

_____

THOUGHTS ABOUT YOUR INFERTILITY

Read the following list of thoughts and feelings that have occurred for other people struggling with infertility. Have you experienced some, all or none of these? Whatever your emotional experience, know that you are not alone in dealing with these struggles, thoughts and emotions. When reading through the list, think about if you have experienced the same thought and how you dealt with it.

Self-blame/guilt: "This is my fault." "It's *my* body that's not working properly, not his." "I must have done something wrong to make this happen to me."

Sense of loss: "All of my hopes and dreams for having a family are gone." "I feel barren and empty."

Anxiety and lack of control: "I feel like I have no control over whether I'm able to have a baby and I'm worried that it will never happen."

Confusion/feeling overwhelmed: "Why is this happening to me?" "I can't make sense of all these treatment options and medications."

Fear of failure: "What if it never happens? What will happen to me? To my relationship with my partner? What will we do?" "I feel like a failure as a woman because I can't get pregnant."

Sadness/depression/hopelessness: "If I can't even do what comes naturally to most women (even those who don't want babies), I'm worthless." "Things will never change."

Social isolation: "I'm alone in this. No one understands what I'm going through."

Social avoidance: "I don't want to see anyone. I don't want to have to answer questions about how it's going and how I'm doing." "I don't want to see looks of pity."

Anger/resentment/sense of unfairness: "Why is this happening to me? Why can *she* get pregnant when I can't?" "Look at that woman mistreating their child, why was she able to have a baby, but not me?"

Numbness: "I feel exhausted by all of this." "I feel empty." "I feel lost."

Difficulty concentrating: "All I think about all day is my inability to have a baby. I can't focus on anything else."

Change in appetite: "I don't feel like eating." "All I do is eat because I'm stressed and upset all the time." "I eat to fill the internal void."

Strained interpersonal relationships: "This infertility has come between me and my partner." "I can't talk to my family about this." "They don't get it."

Loss of interest in previously enjoyable activities/social occasions: "Nothing seems fun to me anymore."

Choose from the list above (or from your own experience) and write down the thoughts that are familiar to you.

_____

_____

_____

_____

Now write down how you manage these thoughts and feelings.

_____

_____

_____

_____

Your feelings and experiences are completely valid and typical for someone dealing with infertility. However, that doesn't mean you have to treat them as facts. They are beliefs and thoughts that you can challenge to lift some of the burden and feel better or more optimistic. Furthermore, there are steps you can take to help you improve your mood and outlook.

CHALLENGING YOUR THOUGHTS

Now that you've identified your thoughts, take the time to explore them. Choose one thought you wrote and rewrite it here:

_____

The following process will help you develop an alternative thought/self-statement to challenge the anxiety-producing or depressing thought. For example, you have a distress-induced thought such as, "This is my fault." Find an alternative way to think about your situation. One alternative may be, "PCOS is a medical condition that many women have." Another might be, "It's not my fault that I have it." Again, another interpretation might be, "There are things I can do and medications I can take to help." Can you think of an alternative thought or interpretation? Write it down here:

_____

_____

_____

Next, choose an action that is associated with your new self-statement. In other words, think about what you can do about the thoughts and feelings you have. For example, "I will collaborate with my treatment team and support network to get though this and have the child I've always wanted." What actions could you take about the thoughts you're having?

_____

_____

_____

Try this exercise again, but this time, challenge other thoughts.

1. Distress-inducing thought:

_____

_____

_____

Alternative thought/self-statement:

_____

_____

_____

_____

Action:

_____

_____

_____

_____

2. Distress-inducing thought:

_____

_____

_____

Alternative thought/self-statement:

_____

_____

_____

_____

Action:

_____

_____

_____

_____

POKED AND PRODDED:
THE IMPROMPTU BLOOD DONOR

The good news about PCOS and infertility: Several medical interventions are available to facilitate fertility and pregnancy. Deciding which option is appropriate for you (see Treatment Options in this chapter) is a matter of discussion with your treatment team, your partner, and recognizing what feels comfortable for you. To determine the possible medical interventions, as well as the best timing for fertilization, your doctors will test your blood frequently to monitor your hormone levels. Doctors are looking for the appropriate amount and ratio of hormones, including: follicle stimulating hormone (FSH), luteinizing hormone (LH), estrogen and progesterone (see Chapter 1). Because hormone levels vary at different stages of the cycle (and we know the cycles of women with PCOS are particularly irregular), frequent testing is needed. In addition to these blood tests, you may also have a transvaginal ultrasound. This procedure is typically done by inserting a probe into the vagina, which uses sound waves to produce a visual image on a monitor. Practitioners use the transvaginal ultrasound to measure the size of the follicle in which the egg is held. As the egg develops, the follicle size increases. Ovulation typically occurs when the follicle is between 1.8 and 2.5 centimeters. Along with the blood tests, the transvaginal ultrasound helps monitor the ovulatory cycle more precisely and is useful to determine timing for intercourse or insemination.

This translates into frequent appointments, blood draws, poking and prodding as well as the emotional ups and downs that occur with each visit. You may start to feel like an involuntary blood donor! This can be particularly difficult for women with needle phobias. While the transvaginal ultrasound is painless, the procedure can be emotionally uncomfortable. You may initially feel particularly exposed, intruded upon or vulnerable. Due to multiple exposures and experiences, these emotions will likely diminish over time.

Many women have said the results of testing become the barometer of how they feel for the day. Because you have no control over your hormone levels or follicular growth, your mood and functioning can also feel out of your control. And because you go for blood draws so frequently, you may start to feel like your life completely revolves around appointments. To regain some semblance of control and a sense of normalcy, try to schedule your appointments for the same time each day and create a routine around the appointment. Consider the appointment a time for self-care. For example, schedule some time near the appointment to read the paper, grab a cup of coffee or call a trusted friend, family member or your partner to cheer you up, give you support or provide a diversion. Take a walk or window shop, if you find these activities relaxing for you. You may be working or have other obligations that constantly get shifted around to make your frequent appointments. This can be particularly distressing if you decide not to divulge your fertility treatment with others, such as your boss or colleagues, thereby requiring a seemingly endless stream of excuses and/or significant schedule juggling. For those of you in this situation, your "routine" or "self-care time" may be limited, but do what you can to include this important strategy.

Write down ideas for "self-care time" following your appointments:

_____

_____

_____

_____

SEX ON A SCHEDULE

The medical interventions used to promote your fertility will likely target stimulating ovulation. When the blood draws and/or transvaginal ultrasound show you are ovulating, your doctors will suggest you have intercourse within a certain time period following your appointment (typically within 24 to 36 hours). While this is phenomenal news, it certainly can change the approach, sense of spontaneity and feelings that are usually associated with sex. Having sex to coordinate with ovulation may feel "medical-ized," "scheduled" or forced.

Initially, you and your partner may experience the sense of awkwardness that comes with your first sexual encounter, even if you have had a healthy sexual relationship for years. With potentially multiple attempts at becoming pregnant, you or your partner may feel that sex has become "an obligation" or "a job" rather than an enjoyable, intimate activity that brings you both closer together and is physically and emotionally satisfying. In addition, what was once an event that was shared only between you and your partner, now feels public. The doctors and nurses at the office know you'll be having sex that evening, as do potentially others who are aware of your fertility treatment. There's nothing like having your mother give you a cheerleading "good luck tonight, honey" after she's called to check in on how your appointment went that morning!

While approaching your sex-on-a-schedule scenario with a sense of humor may help, the process can be incredibly exhausting and demoralizing. A sense of humor can be hard to muster when dealing with frequent doctor's appointments, lack of results and medications that induce ovulation and cause mood instability, bloating and cramping. These are not the optimal conditions for putting you "in the mood"! Open lines of communication with your partner are essential. Provide validation for each other in how you're feeling and how difficult the process can be at times. If possible, attempt to discover new ways to stimulate your partner and encourage him to do the same for you. Falling into the trap of viewing sex as "insemination" is easy. Try not to overlook foreplay for the sake of expediency and accomplishing "the job" of insemination. To prevent this transmutation of sex from intercourse to insemination have a healthy sexual relationship at other times during the month when pregnancy is not likely. Finally, give yourself and your partner empathy by recognizing the stressful conditions under which you're now placed. Reassure each other that this change in your sexual relationship is temporary.

Write down how you are feeling about sex right now:

_____

_____

_____

_____

Share these feelings with your partner and ask him for support. Ask him how he is feeling about the process as well.

Write down questions or suggestions you have for your partner that might open the lines of communication and provide a more positive, less forced experience:

_____

_____

_____

_____

TREATMENT OPTIONS

Clomiphene Citrate (Brand names Clomid®, Serophene®). For women with PCOS, the typical cause of infertility is anovulation (defined as a condition in which a woman rarely or never ovulates). Therefore, medications to stimulate ovulation are the primary treatment option. Clomiphene Citrate (CC), the most commonly prescribed ovulation drug, works by causing the pituitary gland to secrete higher levels of Follicle Stimulating Hormone (FSH), which leads to follicular growth in the ovaries. These follicles contain the eggs. As the follicles mature, they secrete estrogen. If the medication is working properly, approximately one week after the final CC tablet is taken, the pituitary gland becomes hypersensitive to Gonadotropin Releasing Hormone (GnRH), which leads to the release of Luteinizing Hormone (LH). The LH surge is the stimulus for ovulation to occur and the mature follicle releases the egg. For many women with PCOS, once the egg is released, the remaining steps to getting pregnant require no further medical intervention.

A typical therapeutic dose of CC is 50mg (in tablet form) and is taken for five consecutive days starting early in the menstrual cycle, usually day 2, 3, 4 or 5. If you don't menstruate, your doctor will likely prescribe a form of progesterone to induce menstruation, prior to initiating CC treatment. To determine whether CC was successful in inducing ovulation, your serum progesterone level will be checked and/or a transvaginal ultrasound will be administered between days 14 and 18. If ovulation does not occur at 50mg, your doctor may decide to increase the dosage of CC. Anywhere from four to six cycles of CC is recommended before attempting other medications to induce ovulation. If the tests reveal ovulation, your doctor will recommend having intercourse and will provide an optimal window of time for insemination. CC will induce ovulation for approximately 80% of properly selected women. Success rates for pregnancy are about 40% to 45% within six cycles. Beyond six cycles, success rates drop considerably. At this point, you should speak with your treatment team about alternative (or additional) medications and/or procedures.

Side effects of CC are relatively common, but generally mild. Typical side effects include nausea, breast tenderness and mood changes. Hot flashes occur among 10% of women taking CC. Blurred or double vision and severe headaches are rare and should be discussed with your doctor immediately if you experience them. All side effects typically dissipate when you stop treatment. Women taking CC have a 10% chance of having twins. The chance of having triplets and beyond is rare.

Intrauterine Insemination. CC can reduce the quantity of cervical mucus, while increasing its thickness, making it a potential barrier for sperm. If this happens to you, your doctor may recommend intrauterine insemination (IUI) in conjunction with your ovulation drugs. This procedure is timed to coincide with ovulation. Your partner will be asked to produce the semen specimen. Typically, he is requested to refrain from ejaculation from one to three days prior to producing the specimen. The semen is then "washed" or the sperm is separated from other elements of the semen and gathered into a smaller, more concentrated volume. This will likely be done on-site, and can take anywhere from 20 to 60 minutes, depending on the technique used to process the semen. The specimen is placed into a thin, sterilized, soft catheter and ready for insemination. A speculum, like one used during a gynecological exam, is placed in the vagina and your cervix is gently cleansed. Your doctor will insert the catheter in the vagina and release the sperm into your uterine cavity. Your doctor may allow you to remain lying down for a few minutes after the insemination.

If the idea of your conception being "artificial" is distressing to you, have sex following the IUI. Some doctors recommend this as well, to take advantage of a known ovulation period. Success rates for IUI are approximately 15% to 20% per cycle and vary based on a number of factors, such as your age, type of ovarian stimulation, motility of sperm, among others. Typically, trying an alternative form of treatment is recommended if you've gone through four to six cycles of IUI without success.

Side effects of IUI are generally rare. Some minor level of vaginal discomfort may occur, similar to your annual pap smear. Some women report cramping, although this may be related more to ovulation than the procedure itself. Some spotting may occur due to minor injury to the cervix during insemination. Infection may result from unsterilized supplies (although this is an unlikely scenario given today's standards of sterilization and hygiene in labs and offices) or from the semen itself. The chances of the latter are also low, given your partner would likely have been tested for a sexually-transmitted disease (STD) at the start of your fertility treatment. If you are using a sperm donor, choose a facility with a high degree of oversight and monitoring of the sperm and sperm donors.

In Vitro Fertilization. If CC or CC in conjunction with IUI does not result in pregnancy, your doctors may recommend moving on to In Vitro Fertilization (IVF). IVF involves eggs being fertilized by sperm in a laboratory dish and transferred to the uterus, where the fertilized egg(s) may implant in the uterine lining. IVF includes several steps, including: ovarian stimulation, egg retrieval, fertilization, embryo culture and embryo transfer. Each is described briefly here. For a more comprehensive explanation, please see The American Society for Reproductive Medicine's *Assisted Reproductive Technologies: A Guide for Patients* (www.asrm.org/ Patients/patientbooklets/ART.pdf).

Ovarian stimulation. Because you have likely tried CC for ovarian stimulation without success, your doctors may prescribe an injectable medication to hyperstimulate your ovaries. Injectable medications to stimulate ovulation include:

- Follicle Stimulating Hormone (FSH) (Brand names: Follistim™, Gonal-F ®, Bravelle™)
- Human Menopausal Gonadotropins (hMG) (Brand names: Humegon™, Repronex™, Menopur®)
- Luteinizing Hormone (LH) (Brand name: Luveris®)

The goal of hyperstimulation is to mature multiple eggs in the ovaries. Multiple eggs are stimulated because some will not fertilize or will show abnormal development after fertilization. Because timing in IVF is crucial, follicular growth in your ovaries will be monitored by transvaginal ultrasound. You may also undergo blood tests to measure your hormonal response to the medications. When the follicles are ready, you will be given an hCG injection (Human Chorionic Gonadotrophin). hCG is an injectable medication that replaces the natural LH surge and causes the final stage of egg maturation (so the eggs are capable of being fertilized).

Egg retrieval. Usually somewhere between 34 and 36 hours after the hCG injection, your eggs will be retrieved by a transvaginal ultrasound aspiration, which is a minor surgical procedure that can be performed in your doctor's office. Some form of anesthetic is generally provided. We encourage you to talk to your doctor about options for analgesia. The procedure entails an ultrasound probe being inserted in the vagina to identify the follicles, after which a needle is guided through the vagina and into the follicles. The needle is connected to a suction device, which helps remove the eggs from the follicles. The procedure typically takes less than 30 minutes. Some women may experience cramping, which usually dissipates within 24 hours of the procedure. Because the ovaries enlarge through stimulation and the hCG injection, you may also experience a sense of pressure or fullness.

Fertilization. Once the eggs are retrieved, they are examined. Mature eggs are identified and placed in a special fluid or IVF culture medium. Sperm are then placed in the IVF culture medium with the mature eggs (oocytes) and transferred to an incubator overnight. Fertilization occurs when the sperm and egg fuse. Approximately 40% to 70% of mature eggs will fertilize.

Embryo culture. Embryo culture refers to the growth of the embryo in the laboratory dish. The fertilized egg divides to become a two- to four-cell embryo by the second day after egg retrieval. By the third day, it is a six-to-ten cell embryo. By day five, the placenta and fetal tissues of the embryo begin to separate within a fluid filled cavity that has developed. Embryos can be transferred back to the uterus any time between one and six days after egg retrieval.

Embryo transfer. The final step of IVF is the transfer of the embryo in the uterus. While no anesthesia is necessary, you may choose to have a mild sedative. A transfer catheter containing one or more embryos (suspended in a drop of IVF culture medium) is guided through your cervix and into the uterine cavity. Your doctor then places the embryo(s) in your uterus via the syringe located at the end of the catheter. The number of embryos transferred is based on guidelines developed by the American Society for Reproductive Medicine. You and your doctor will have discussed these guidelines and your decision prior to the IVF process. You may also have the option for cryopreservation, which is the process of freezing embryos for future transfer. Frozen embryos can be stored for several years. However, not all embryos survive the process of cryopreservation and future thawing.

Decisions regarding how many embryos you transferred at one time and cryopreservation are weighty decisions that entail a variety of factors, including family-building plans and dreams, religious and moral beliefs and odds ratio scenarios (i.e., the odds of getting pregnant given the number of embryos transferred). Some of these factors may be in conflict. Given the emotional roller coaster you've endured thus far, making a "rational" decision may feel overwhelming and unattainable. Give yourself and your partner patience and empathy during this decision-making process.

What are the main issues and factors involved in your decision-making process? Include the pros and cons of your options as well as your hopes, concerns and feelings about this process. Discuss this with your partner and your treatment team.

Pros	Cons

Side effects of IVF may include cramping after egg retrieval and/or embryo transfer. This typically dissipates within a day. Ovarian hyperstimulation syndrome (OHSS) occurs in nearly 30% of women who are taking injectable medications for ovarian stimulation. OHSS takes place when the ovaries become swollen and painful due to hyperstimulation. Fluid can accumulate in the abdominal cavity and cause bloating, nausea and/or lack of appetite. These symptoms are typically managed by a temporary reduction in activity and over-the-counter pain medications. The chance of a multiple pregnancy is increased when more than one embryo is transferred.

Success rates of IVF vary from clinic to clinic and are based on a number of factors, including the types of patients they treat and treatment approaches they use. You can find recent success rates for your IVF program through these websites:

- Centers for Disease Control and Prevention at www.cdc.gov/art.
- Society for Assisted Reproductive Technology at www.sart.org.

Acupuncture

Acupuncture is a form of non-Western medicine that can be beneficial for restoring ovulation and increasing the chances of getting pregnant. The goal of this drug-free intervention is to restore energy flow, or "chi" within the body, based on the idea that the blocked energy at more than 2,000 acupuncture points in the body can result in illness, pain or injury. The process involves placing hair-thin needles just under the skin at specific points of the body to relieve the blockage of energy. For chronic conditions such as PCOS, a series of sessions may be recommended. Several studies have been conducted on the benefit of acupuncture for infertility. For example, one study found that 43% of women who had acupuncture before and after IVF treatments became pregnant, whereas only 26% of age-matched women who had IVF alone conceived. Other studies have shown improvements in ovulation and ovulatory cycles. Therefore, you may want to discuss acupuncture as a complementary treatment with your partner and your treatment team.

Overwhelmed by science

The section you just read provides a significant amount of information about medication and treatment options. In conjunction with information provided by your treatment team, you may have more questions than answers. The intense emotional experience associated with fertility treatment, the multiple appointments and vast amount of medical information, plus the experience of getting good or bad news may make processing this information while in your doctor's office quite difficult. Be patient and empathic with yourself. During doctor appointments, bring your partner, family member or a trusted friend, who may be able to hear and anticipate questions in the moment.

In addition, write down a few questions you have before your next visit.

_____

_____

_____

_____

Keeping a small journal or diary that includes dates of doctor's appointments, timelines, recommendations from doctors, medications and dosages and other medical information (including your responses to various treatments) may be helpful. If this is too overwhelming to manage, ask your partner to help you keep track, either by keeping a journal or entering information together.

THE WAITING ROOM WHO'S WHO

Through the many appointments, you will become quite familiar with your doctor's waiting room. Waiting rooms elicit a variety of emotions for women struggling with infertility. It can be a place of hope for the work you're doing may result in a pregnancy this month or it can be a place of anxiety, where worry thoughts and memories of past disappointments are intense and palpable. Waiting rooms might also be a place of frustration, especially if your doctor tends to run behind schedule or it may be a place of relief: "All these other women are struggling too. I'm not alone." If fertility treatments continue for more than a year, it may be a place of demoralization or numbness: "Here we are again." You may experience all, some or none of these emotions.

Another commonly held experience is the tendency to look around the waiting room with curiosity and wonder. "Where is that couple in this process?" "What treatment is she getting?" "They're going through *that* door, they must be getting that treatment." This may be coupled with a desire to start talking to others, "Well, we all know why we're here… there's no reason to ignore it!" This sense of curiosity and attempts to figure out other patients' issues or treatments is not voyeuristic but a desire to connect. Particularly in times of stress or anxiety, we have a natural tendency to seek out similarly struggling individuals to feel less alone, less anxious and more "normal." Don't feel guilty or ashamed of your "who's who" game. Plan in advance what you'd like to do during your visits to make them less stressful, frustrating or anxiety-provoking for you. You may want to connect with your partner, read, practice deep-breathing, catch up on the news, finish some paperwork, knit or simply sit in silence and meditate.

Write down a few things you can do while in the waiting room:

_____

_____

_____

_____

Babies, babies everywhere!

At a time when a considerable amount of mental, emotional and physical energy are being channeled into having a baby, you may see everyone around you is getting pregnant and having babies. Part of this may be reality, after all your friends are likely to be a similar age. However, your intense and sometimes singular focus on pregnancy may also increase your sensitivity to baby-related information that you previously overlooked. Children in the food store, shows and commercials on television, pictures on colleagues' desks or the news of a friend-of-a-friend-of-a-friend becoming pregnant may not have registered or only slightly registered in the past. Now, however, these may be the *only* things that register. Daily reminders of your desire to have a child and your difficulty in doing so can increase your feelings of hopelessness, depression, anxiety and isolation. You may experience feelings of resentment or jealousy toward loved ones and valued friends who get pregnant. You may choose not to attend events such as baby showers or other social gatherings where pregnancy and children will likely be the main topic of conversation. This sense of dejection or isolation may wax and wane. One day you spend an enjoyable afternoon with a friend and her baby and the next day need to dash out of the grocery store in tears when you see a mother with her baby. Be patient with yourself.

Your feelings of resentment toward friends and family and your decisions to decline invitations to social events, while self-protective, may generate feelings of guilt. Thoughts such as "I *should* be happy for her. She wanted a baby badly, too" or "I *ought* to go to that baby shower, she would go to mine." If ever there were a time to throw out the rigid guilt- and shame-inducing "should's and ought's" that time is now! Give yourself empathy for the distressing situation you're currently experiencing and engage in some much needed self-care. Recognize that your family and friends will understand, but they're not mind-readers. Communicate with them (to the degree that you feel comfortable) regarding your experi- ence. They may be an important source of support for you. Nevertheless, everyone knows someone who can't seem to understand how their joy might be your heartache. A clear and concise statement from you can go a long way to decreasing your stress (even if it takes a few repetitions for that person to get it) or ask your partner to communicate to your network on your behalf.

Practice here. What can you say to a friend or family member when declining an invitation?

_____

_____

_____

_____

What are some self-care activities you can do instead of attending a social event?

_____

_____

_____

_____

Rallying the troops or keeping them at bay: your support network

Your support network, including your partner, family members and friends, are an impor- tant part of the treatment process and may be integral in helping you through it. You may be thinking to yourself, "This is a private matter" or "I'm always the rock." We encourage you to challenge this self-talk and open yourself up to appropriate support of others around you. We say *appropriate* because we recognize that you may need different people at different times. For example, you may need someone to distract you, make you laugh or cry with. More typi- cally, you may need to rally the troops and have different people serve the various functions that meet your needs. While your support system loves and cares for you, they are not mind readers. Help them help you by telling them how they can be the most supportive.

Identify the members of your support network:

_____

_____

_____

_____

Now list how each one can be supportive to you:

_____

_____

_____

_____

We also recognize that there's a time to "keep them at bay." That is, you may need some time to yourself to process this experience. This is completely appropriate and usually necessary. However, understanding the difference between choosing to be alone to decompress, choosing to be alone to avoid others, your experience, emotions and functioning (i.e., isolating yourself) is important. The former is health-promoting while the latter can be harmful and seem counter-productive to getting pregnant. Often loved ones don't recognize the difference. You may experience some of the well intentioned but overwhelming phone calls, offers to talk, uninvited drop-ins or requests for dinner.

Write down a few ways to comfortably but affirmatively communicate when you're feeling besieged.

_____

_____

_____

_____

If you don't have a support system or find yourself isolating and withdrawing from others or your support network isn't enough, seek the support of a therapist who is trained in fertility issues to help you find strategies. This therapist can become an invaluable component of your treatment team and serve in a variety of functions, such as: helping to gather and sort through information, strengthening coping strategies to manage the stress, anxiety and depression; preparing for and coping with medical procedures; reducing the strain on your support system (or helping you set appropriate boundaries with them); exploring alternative family-building options; processing the losses associated with infertility; improving communication with others; and continuing to build a fulfilling life. To find an experienced therapist near you, visit:

- The Mental Health Professional Group of the American Society of Reproductive Medicine (ASRM) at www.asrm.org/mhpg.
- The American Psychological Association (APA) at www.apa.org.
- RESOLVE: The National Infertility Association at www.resolve.org.

MORE THAN A SPERM DONOR: YOUR PARTNER'S EXPERIENCE

Couples who have gone through fertility treatment often report an increased closeness, bond or sense of shared goals and dreams in their relationship. However, like you, your partner carries with him his own set of expectations and hopes for the family you both want. Since your partner is certainly more than a simple sperm donor when it comes to fertility treatment this process may take an emotional toll on him as well. Your partner will experience a range of emotions regarding the medications, procedures and results you both face. Understand what thoughts and feelings your partner may experience.

Many partners report a sense of helplessness. While some men have a natural tendency to problem-solve, your partner has little capacity to "fix" your ovulation cycle or the thickness of your uterine lining. Your partner may have a difficult time watching you undergo a variety of emotionally painful and sometimes physically uncomfortable procedures. He may also feel powerless to "take away" the emotional distress you experience. Since helplessness is one of the more intolerable emotions to men, he may show frustration or anger instead. If you find that you and your partner are getting irritable with each other more easily during this process, you are not alone. In addition to helplessness, your partner may feel a lack of control over the process and outcome. In the same way he can't "fix" things, he also can't control them. This is a distressing feeling to carry, particularly when you are in pain. While your job is not to "fix" his helplessness, communicating with him about his feelings and finding ways that he can participate and gain a sense of control will be beneficial. For example, you may decide that he could be the primary "researcher" and gather information on the medications and procedures recommended by your treatment team. Alternatively, your partner could plan or accompany you to one of your activities to reduce your stress level.

Discuss with your partner his feelings about your current treatments and ways you might find him to be helpful. Write a few ideas here:

_____

_____

_____

_____

In addition to a sense of helplessness and a lack of control, worry and uncertainty about the future are common emotions that partners report. Partners may worry about your well-being, the risks and benefits of various procedures, the financial strain of long-term fertility treatments, the outcome of the next cycle and the uncertainty about the future. Because they may not be able to make every appointment, they are sometimes insulated from the process. While this may sound like a protective factor, it can occasionally lead to feelings of uncertainty, confusion and a sense of being cut off. Like you, your partner may feel overwhelmed by the medical information. After all, he doesn't have the years of experience with the female anatomy that you do! However, just like you, your partner needs coping strategies to help manage his stress level.

Encourage your partner to identify activities that reduce stress and distress in his life. Write them down here. This way, if you find your partner is stressed or you seem to be irritable toward each other, you can encourage him to engage in one of these activities.

_____

_____

_____

_____

Note: Your partner may experience feelings of anxiety or depression as a result of this process. He, too, could benefit from therapy with an experienced mental health provider.

Finally, try to remember that you're still a strong and happy couple with an active life! Try not to let your fertility treatments define you, your activities or your lifestyle. Continue your date nights and travel plans, commemorate major milestones and exciting events. Cherish your respective accomplishments and explore new facets of each other. Celebrate strong friendships and loving family. Continue to grow together in your rich and fulfilling lives.

CHAPTER 9

MANAGING PCOS

MANAGING your PCOS is extremely important. If left unchecked, PCOS can lead to further medical complications later in life. The following are a list of medical conditions that women with PCOS tend to experience. The good news: All of these conditions are preventable or treatable by adopting a healthy regimen of eating and exercise. Along with discussing the most common medical conditions that women with PCOS can develop, this chapter explains which health care professional manages what part of your treatment.

BEYOND PCOS: OTHER MEDICAL CONDITIONS

Dyslipidemia occurs when blood cholesterol levels (total cholesterol, LDL, HDL, or triglycerides) are abnormal. Maintaining healthy blood lipids levels are needed to decrease your risk of cardiovascular disease, stroke and heart attack. Triglycerides or LDL (the "bad" cholesterol) can build up and form plaque in the walls of the arteries. Narrowing of the arteries prevents adequate blood flow to the heart and brain resulting in stroke or heart attack. Usually women with PCOS have high levels of triglycerides (the blood storage form of fat) and low HDL (the "good" cholesterol).

A healthy eating and exercise plan may prevent and treat dyslipidemia. HDL (the "good cholesterol") works to rid the body of cholesterol. Medications in combination with diet and exercise may also be effective at improving cholesterol levels.

Hypertension, also known as "the silent killer" is the term for elevated blood pressure. Because there are no symptoms, many people don't know they have hypertension unless they get their blood pressure checked regularly. Uncontrolled hypertension can lead to stroke, heart attack, heart failure or kidney failure. An optimal blood pressure is < 120/80.

Because most women with PCOS are overweight, they are at high risk for hypertension. A low-sodium diet, rich in fruits and vegetables, regular exercise and medication, if needed, offer the best chance to reduce blood pressure.

Diabetes is classified by two different types. Type 1 is typically diagnosed in childhood. Because the pancreas is unable to produce insulin, individuals must inject themselves with it to survive.

Type 2 diabetes, the most common form of diabetes, is diagnosed when blood glucose levels remain high in the blood. The body either can't produce enough insulin to meet the need or the insulin receptors are resistant and don't respond to the insulin available. Consequences of prolonged high blood sugar are cardiovascular disease, stroke and nerve damage. Type 2 diabetes is diagnosed when a fasting blood glucose reaches 126 milligrams per deciliter (mg/dL) or higher. Symptoms include increased thirst and hunger, fatigue, increased urination, weight loss or blurred vision. The best treatment for type 2 diabetes is a combination of exercise, diet and medication. Most individuals with type 2 diabetes will need to monitor their blood sugar levels daily.

Women with PCOS are at high risk for type 2 diabetes in the long-term as insulin receptors can become resistant over time and eventually ignore insulin. Type 2 diabetes is preventable in women with PCOS who adopt a healthy eating and exercise regime and, if prescribed, comply with their medications. Metformin® (glucophage), a common PCOS medication, is also prescribed for type 2 diabetes and may decrease the risk of diabetes in PCOS.

Hypothyroidism or underactive thyroid is a condition in which your thyroid gland doesn't produce enough of hormones, upsetting the normal balance of chemical reactions in your body. Common symptoms of hypothyroidism include fatigue, dry skin, weight gain and difficulties losing weight. According to the Mayo Clinic, untreated hypothyroidism can cause obesity, joint pain, infertility and heart disease.

The good news: a simple blood test called thyroid-stimulating hormone (TSH) can diagnose hypothyroidism. Treatment of the disease, a pill containing synthetic thyroid hormone, is usually simple, safe and effective once the proper dosage is established.

Based on symptoms of PCOS, physicians may request blood tests to rule out hypothyroidism. If you suspect you may have this condition, please consult with your physician.

Metabolic syndrome is a collection of health risks that increase the chance of developing heart disease, stroke or diabetes. You must have at least three of the following conditions to have metabolic syndrome: Elevated blood pressure, low HDL, elevated triglycerides, excess insulin, elevated fasting glucose and excess weight in the mid-section. The best treatment for metabolic syndrome is a combination of diet, exercise and possibly medications.

Obstructive sleep apnea (OSA) occurs when you stop breathing for 10 seconds or more at least five times an hour, decreasing oxygen in the blood while sleeping. Causes of OSA include excess weight and high testosterone levels. Signs of OSA include snoring with intermittent pauses, excessive daytime sleepiness, gasping and choking during sleep, fragmented and non-refreshing sleep, decreased sex drive and morning headaches. Consequences of OSA may include elevated blood pressure, higher risk for a heart disease and heart attack, insulin resistance and metabolic syndrome. Treatment for OSA is a called Continuous Positive

Airway Pressure (CPAP) which provides a mask to be worn during sleep to increase oxygen intake. Not sleeping on your back is also recommended to keep your airway open.

Non-alcoholic fatty liver disease occurs when fat accumulates in the liver of a person who drinks little or no alcohol. Non-alcoholic fatty liver disease is associated with obesity, insulin resistance, high blood pressure, diabetes, elevated cholesterol and high triglyceride levels. Early stages of this disease may show no symptoms. The main symptoms are fatigue and a dull pain in the upper right abdomen. Eating a high fat diet does not cause non-alcoholic fatty liver disease. One theory suggests fat accumulates because the liver has difficulty converting fat into an easy eliminating form. Medications that pass though the liver may also contribute the disease. It can be detected and monitored by liver function tests (also known as LFTs) and is often treated by medications and weight loss.

Are you a distorted eater?

Many women with PCOS struggle with eating issues as they use food and/or weight-controlling behaviors to cope with intense feelings and emotions. Anxiety and depression, very common among the PCOS population, may contribute to eating issues also. In addition, PCOS is associated with many dermatological issues that can affect body image, like having extra weight around your middle or excessive hair growth or acne. Not surprisingly, women with PCOS struggle with their body image and are more prone to develop distorted eating methods such as emotional eating or eating disorders (see below). (For more on body image please see Chapter 6 which is devoted to this topic.)

Emotional eating is eating food when you are not physically hungry. People who engage in emotional eating are usually doing so to self-soothe or comfort themselves. For example, if you are having a bad day, you may turn to your favorite comfort food to feel better. Or maybe you are feeling very overwhelmed and eating your favorite candy is a quick and tasty way to calm yourself. For many, emotional eating is established in childhood and continues into adulthood. However, it is only a temporary fix that may lead to weight gain, making life seem even more stressful. If you are eating and not hungry, you're giving your body more energy (calories) than it needs. This can worsen insulin levels and hamper weight loss efforts.

Eating disorders. There are three main types of eating disorders: binge eating disorder, bulimia and anorexia nervosa. Binge eating disorder is when someone eats large amounts of food, more than what someone would typically consume, in an out-of-control manner. The binge episodes, mostly done in secret, must occur at least two days a week for six months to meet the diagnostic criteria for binge eating disorder.

Bulimia nervosa is when someone will binge eat and purge by vomiting, taking laxatives or engaging in extreme exercise to get rid of the food or calories. Behaviors must occur twice a week for three months or longer to meet criteria for bulimia nervosa.

Anorexia nervosa is when someone sees themselves as fat even when they are underweight. People with anorexia will fear food and eat little amounts. They may engage in compulsive exercise and other methods to control their weight. Due to their low body weight, women with anorexia will lack menstrual cycles.

Eating disorders can be life-threatening and get worse over time. Anyone who struggles with emotional eating or has an eating disorder needs professional treatment involving a therapist, dietitian and physician.

Mental health concerns

With out of balance hormones, erratic periods, general frustration with having PCOS and dealing with its symptoms, women with PCOS tend to experience more mental health disorders than other women. Anxiety (which is different than occasional worry) is seen in women who are overly concerned about weight, shape, body image and social situations. Anxiety disorders can be successfully treated. If you think you struggle with anxiety, seek the assistance of a professional.

Some women with PCOS may also experience episodes of depression. While many people feel "sad" or "blue," clinical depression is qualitatively different and lasts longer, and may be classified as depressive disorder or bipolar depression. If you think you might be struggling with depression, you must seek the guidance of a professional.

Use the space provided to write notes or questions you have to discuss with your doctor:

_____

_____

_____

_____

_____

_____

_____

Let's go team!

Depending on the symptoms, the treatment of PCOS may involve different medical specialties: Gynecology, fertility experts, dermatology, endocrinology, and nutrition to name a few. Below are definitions of different health care professionals who may assist you in your treatment. Members of your treatment team should communicate with each other to best support your care. Since you are also a member of your treatment team (an important member!), keep a journal listing the medications and supplements you are taking. Be sure to include the appropriate dosage and accompanying lab results. Take the journal to each appointment. You might also want to record your experiences at each appointment as well as what you and your treatment provider discussed. A list of "Resources for PCOS," in the appendix can help you to locate health providers in your area.

Endocrinologist. Clinical endocrinologists are specialists in the care and evaluation of patients with hormonal disorders such as thyroid disease, PCOS and diabetes.

Obstetrician/Gynecologist. An obstetrician is a physician who specializes in the management of pregnancy and labor. A gynecologist is a physician specializes in the female reproductive system. An obstetrician/gynecologist is a physician who provides medical and surgical care to women and has particular expertise in pregnancy, childbirth and disorders of the reproductive system, such as PCOS.

Reproductive Endocrinologist. These are Obstetrician-Gynecologists with advanced education, research and professional skills in reproductive hormones and infertility. These physicians treat reproductive disorders that affect children, women and men as well as infertility in men and women. These specialists can help you become pregnant and/or manage your PCOS. Reproductive endocrinologists often monitor your first trimester of pregnancy and then transfer you to an obstetrician for the remainder of your pregnancy.

General Internist. These physicians are experts in health promotion, disease prevention, diagnosis and treatment of chronic illness. They are not limited to one type of medical problem. General internists, such as a primary care physician, often care for patients during the duration of their adult lives, providing an opportunity for the physician and patient to establish a long-term professional relationship. General internists can subspecialize in other medical fields such as endocrinology, adolescent medicine and women's health.

Registered Dietitian (RD). Dietitians are trained to provide reliable and objective nutrition information and will assist you in making the appropriate changes to your eating to improve your health. RDs help you understand PCOS as well as help you to make lasting changes in your eating habits. They will also challenge any distorted thinking you may have around food and help you be a more mindful eater. You may choose to work with a dietitian regularly as a source of support, education and accountability to make changes in your eating.

Dermatologist. A dermatologist specializes in the treatment of skin and treats many PCOS symptoms, including acne, hair growth, balding and acanothis nigricans.

Therapist. A therapist treats psychological problems. You might choose to see a psychiatrist (MD), a psychologist (PhD or Psy.D), a licensed professional counselor (LPC) or a social worker (LCSW). Therapists can help with emotional eating, eating disorders, depression, anxiety, relationship distress, body image issues or stress management. If you're looking for a therapist in your area, ask your doctor for a referral or visit the American Psychological Association's website, www.APA.org.

Write down the current members of your treatment team:

_____   _____

_____   _____

_____   _____

_____   _____

What other health professionals or resources do you need to help you to manage your PCOS?

_____

_____

_____

_____

A list of Resources for PCOS is located in the appendix. Use the space below to write down some providers and resources in your area that you would be interested in seeking support from:

Name   Phone number

_____   _____

_____   _____

_____   _____

_____   _____

_____   _____

_____   _____

_____   _____

_____   _____

You're now on the road to managing your PCOS. The road ahead may be bumpy at times, but with the right tools, information, treatment team and awareness of how to live with PCOS in a healthy way, your life is sure to be full and satisfying. Remember, one out of ten women struggle with PCOS. You are not alone.

GLOSSARY

Acanthosis nigricans – velvety, dark patches usually seen behind the neck, armpits, and genital areas; markers of elevated insulin.

Alopecia – baldness.

Alpha linolenic acid (ALA) – omega-3 fatty acids found in plant foods such as flaxseed, walnuts, and canola oil.

Amenorrhea – absence of menstruation.

Androgens – male hormones such as testosterone and dehydroepiandrosterone sulfate (DHEA-sulfate).

Anovulation – rare or no ovulation.

Clomid Citrate – a fertility medication used to stimulate ovulation.

Cortisol – a stress hormone.

Cryopreservation – the process of freezing embryos for future transfer.

DHEA-sulfate – dehydroepiandrosterone sulfate, an androgen.

Docosahexaenoic acid (DHA) - an omega 3 fatty acid found in fish.

Dyslipidemia – a term for abnormal blood cholesterol levels.

Eicosapentaenoic acid (EPA) - an omega 3 fatty acid found in fish.

Embyro – the early stages of fetal growth, from conception to the eighth week of pregnancy.

Follicle Stimulating Hormone (FSH) – a hormone responsible for egg development.

Ghrelin – a hormone involved in appetite regulation.

Glycemic index – a rate at which a food will increase your insulin levels.

Gonadotropin Releasing Hormone (GnRH) – a hormone that is involved with stimulating ovulation.

HDL – high-density lipoproteins, the "good" cholesterol.

Hirsutism – excessive facial and body hair, usually due to elevated androgens.

Human Chorionic Gonadotrophin (hCG) – an injectable fertility medication that aids in egg maturation.

Hyperandrogenism – elevated levels of androgens.

Hyperinsulinemia – over-production of insulin.

Hypertension – elevated blood pressure.

Hypoglycemia – low blood sugar as evidenced by increased hunger, crankiness, dizziness and nausea.

Hypothyroidism – underactive thyroid gland.

Insulin – a growth hormone that promotes fat storage and assists with blood glucose regulation.

Insulin resistance – condition where insulin receptors on cells don't respond well to insulin resulting in excess insulin.

In Vitro Fertilization (IVF) – a fertility process in which eggs are fertilized by sperm in a laboratory dish and transferred to the uterus.

LDL – low-density lipoproteins, the "bad" cholesterol.

LH/FSH ratio – comparison of luteinizing hormone to follicle-stimulating hormone.

Leptin – a hormone involved in appetite regulation.

Luteinizing Hormone (LH) – a hormone that plays a role in egg maturation and release. Usually in PCOS, LH levels are elevated.

Metabolic Syndrome – a combination of medical conditions that increase the risk of developing heart disease and diabetes. Also known as syndrome X.

Oligomenorrhea – erratic menstrual cycling.

Refined carbohydrates – processed grains that enter bloodstream rapidly. Usually indicated on food labels as "enriched."

Triglycerides – a storage form of fat in your bloodstream.

Type 1 Diabetes – a form of diabetes usually diagnosed in childhood where the pancreas is unable to produce insulin.

Type 2 Diabetes – a form of diabetes in which the body either makes too little insulin or cannot properly use the insulin it makes to convert blood glucose into energy.

Whole grains – intact grains indicated as a first ingredient in ingredient list as 'whole.'

REFERENCES

Chapter 1

Barbierei, R.L. (2003). Metformin for treatment of polycystic ovary syndrome. *Obstetrics and Gynecology, 101,* 785-793.

Dunaif, A., Segal, K.R., Futterweit, W. & Dobrjansky, A. (1989). Profound peripheral insulin resistance, independent of obesity, in polycystic ovary syndrome. *Diabetes,* 38, 1165-1174.

Jakubowicz, D.J, Iuorno, M.J., Jakubowicz, S.,Roberts, K.A., & Nestler, J.E. (2002). Effects of metformin on early pregnancy loss in polycystic ovary syndrome. *Journal of Clinical Endocrinology and Metabolism, 87,* 524-529.

Lego, R.S., Finegood, D., & Dunaif, A. (1998). A fasting glucose to insulin ratio is a useful measure of insulinsensitivity in women with polycystic ovary syndrome. *The Journal of Clinical Endocrinology and Metabolism,* 83, 2694-2698.

Lewy, V.D., Danadian, K, Witchel, S.F., & Arslanian, S. (2001). Early metabolic abnormalities in adolescent girls with polycystic ovarian syndrome. *Journal of Pediatrics,* 138, 38–44.

Lord, J.M., Flight, I.K. & Norman, R.J. (2003). Metformin in polycystic ovary syndrome: Systemic review and meta-analysis. *British Medical Journal, 327,* 951.

Sharma, S., Nestler, J. (2006). Prevention of diabetes and cardiovascular disease in women with PCOS: treatment with insulin sensitizers. *Best Practice Research Clinical Endocrinology and Metabolism,* 20(2), 245-260.

Sherif, K. (1999) Benefits and risks of oral contraceptives. *American Journal of Obstetrics and Gynecology,* 180(6),343-348.

Sherif, K (2007). Understanding PCOS. In. A. Grassi's *The Dietitian's Guide to Polycystic Ovary Syndrome.* Luca Publishing: Haverford, PA.

The Rotterdam ESHRE/ASRM sponsored PCOS consensus workshop group: revised 2003 consensus on diagnostic criteria and long term health risks related to polycystic ovary syndrome. *Fertility and Sterility, 2004,* 81, 19-25.

Zawedzki, J.K. & Dunaif, A. (1992). Diagnostic criteria for polycystic ovary syndrome: towards a rational approach. In: Dunaif A, Givens JR, Haseltine FP, Merriam GR, Eds. *Polycystic ovary syndrome:* Boston: Glasckwell Scientific, 377-384.

Chapter 2

Chavarro, J., Willet, W. & Skerrett, P. (2007) *The Fertility Diet.* McGraw-Hill: New York, NY.

Choose Your Foods: Exchange List for Diabetes (2008). American Dietetic Association: Chicago, IL.

Calder, P.C. (June 2006). "n–3 polyunsaturated fatty acids, inflammation, and inflammatory diseases". American Journal of Clinical Nutrition 83 (6, supplement), 1505S–1519S.

Douglas, C.C., Norris, L.E., Oster, R.A.,Darnell, B.E., Azziz, R. & Gower, B.A .(2006) Difference in dietary intake between women with polycystic ovary syndrome and healthy controls. *Fertility and Sterility,* 86, 411-417.

Marsh, K. & Brand-Miller, J . (2005). The optimal diet for women with polycystic ovary syndrome. *British*

Journal of Nutrition. 94, 154-165.

Moran L.J., Noakes, M., Clifton, M., Tomlisson, L. & Norman, R.J. (2003). Dietary composition in restoring reproductive and metabolic physiology in overweight women with polycystic ovary syndrome. *Journal of Clinical Endocrinology Metabolism*, 88, 812-819.

Stamets, K. (2004). A randomized trial of the effects of two types of short-term hypocaloric diets on weight loss in women with polycystic ovary syndrome. *Fertility and Sterility*, 81(3), 630-637.

Chapter 3

The American Dietetic Association (2007). *The plant sterol story: using food choices to help manage cholesterol.* Nutrition Fact Sheet. www.eatright.org/ada/files/The_Plant_Sterol_Story.pdf.

Anderson, R.A (2005). Polyphenols from cinnamon increase insulin sensitivity: Functional and clinical aspects [abstract]. *Dietary Antioxidants, Trace Elements, Vitamins and Polyphenols*, 4, 154.

Bhathena S.J. (2000). Relationship between fatty acids and the endocrine system. *Biofactors*, 13, 35-39.

Chiu, KC, et al (2004). Hypovitaminosis D is associated with insulin resistance and beta cell dysfunction. *Americal Jouranl of Clinical Nutrition*, 79, 820-825.

He, K., Liu, K., Daviglus, M.L., Morris, S.J. & Loria, C.M. (2006). Magnesium intake and incidence of metabolic syndrome among young adults. *Circulation*, 113, 1675-1682.

Khan, A., Safdar, M., Khan, M., Khan, K. & Anderson,R. (2003). Cinnamon improves glucose and lipids of people with type 2 diabetes. *Diabetes Care*, 26, 3215-3218.

Iuorno, M.J., Jakubowicz, D.J., Baillargeon, J.P. (2002). Effects of d-chiro-inositol in lean women with polycystic ovary syndrome. *Endocrine Practice, 8* (6), 417-423.

Nestler, J., Jakubowicz, D., Reamer, P., Gunn, R.D. & Allen, G. (1999). Ovulatory and metabolic effects of d-chiro inositol in the polycystic ovary syndome. *New England Journal of Medicine*, 340, 1314-1320.

Papaleo, E., Unfer, V., Baillargeon, J.P., et al. (2007). Myo-inositol in patients with polycystic ovary syndrome: A novel method for ovulation induction. *Gynecological Endrocrinology,23* (12), 700-703.

Parker, G., Gibson, N.A., Brotchie, H. & Heruc, G. (2006). Omega-3 fatty acids and mood disorders. *American Journal of Psychiatry*, 163, 969-980.

Thomson, R., Buckley J., Noakes M., Clifton, P.M., Norman, R.J., & Brinkworth, G.D. (2008). The effect of a hypocaloric diet with and without exercise training on body composition, cariometabolic risk profile and reproductive function in overweight and obese women with polycystic ovary syndrome. *The Journal of Clinical Endocrinology and Metabolism, (*93), 3373-3380.

Thys-Jacobs, S., Donovan, D., Papadopoulos, A, Sarrel, P. & Bilezikian, J.P. (1999) Vitamin D and calcium dysregulation in the polycystic ovarian syndrome. *Steroids*, 64(6), 430-435.

Chapter 5

Aldwin, C.M. (2007). *Stress, coping, and development: An Integrative perspective.* Guilford Press: NY.

Brown, A.J. (2004). Depression and insulin resistance: Applications to polycystic ovary syndrome. *Clinical Obstetrics and Gynecology*, 47(3), 592-596.

Epel, E., Lapidus, R., McEwen, B. & Brownell, K. (2001). Stress may add bite to appetite in women: a laboratory study of stress-induced cortisol and eating behavior. Psychoneuroendocrinology *(26)37-49.*

Himelein, M.J., & Thatcher, S.S. (2006b). Polycystic ovary syndrome and mental health: A Review. *Obstetrical and gynecological survey*, 61 (11);723-732.

Kabat-Zinn, J. (1991). Full catastrophe living; Using the wisdom of your body and mind to face stress, pain and illness. Random House: New York, NY.

Linehan, M.M. (1993) Cognitive-Behavioral Treatment of Borderline Personality Disorder. Guilford Press. NY.

Linehan, M. (1993) Skills Training Manual for Treating Borderline Personality Disorder. Guilford Press. NY.

Mattei, S. (2007). Psychological Aspects of Polycystic Ovary Syndrome, In. A. Grassi's *The Dietitian's Guide to*

Polycystic Ovary Syndrome. Luca Publishing: Haverford, PA.

Modell, E., Goldstein, D., Reyes, F.I. (1990). Endocrine and behavioral responses to psychological stress in hyperandrogenic women. *Fertility and Sterility,* 53, 454-459.

Moreira, R O. Marca, K F. Appolinario, J C. &Coutinho, W F. (2007). Increased waist circumference is associated with an increased prevalence of mood disorders and depressive symptoms in obese women. *Eating & Weight Disorders,* 12(1), 35-40.

Okamura F, Tashiro A, Utumi A, et al. (2000). Insulin resistance in patients with depression and its changes during the clinical course of depression: minimal model analysis. *Metabolism,* 49,1255-1260.

Thatcher, S.S. (2000). *Polycystic ovary syndrome: The Hidden Epidemic.* Perspectives Press: Indianapolis, IN.

Tsilchorozidou,T.,Honour, J.W., & Conway, G. S. (2003). Altered cortisol metabolism in Polycystic ovary syndrome: Insulin enhances 5 -reduction but not the elevated adrenal steroid production rates. *The Journal of Clinical Endocrinology and Metabolism,* 88(12), 5907-5913.

Chapter 6

Cash, T.F. (1997). *The Body image workbook: An 8-Step program for learning to like your looks.* New Harbinger, CA.

Clark, L & Tiggeman, M. (2008). Sociocultural and individual psychological predictors of body image in young girls: A Prospective study. *Developmental Psychology,* 44 (4), 1124-1134.

Himelein, M.J., & Thatcher, S.S. (2006). Depression and body image among women with Polycystic Ovary Syndrome. *Journal of Health psychology,* 11(4) 613-625.

Jones, D.C. (2004). Body image among adolescent girls and boys: A longitudinal study. *Developmental Psychology,* 40, 823-835.

Lipton M.G., Sherr, L.,& Elford, J. (2006). Women living with facial hair: The psychological and behavioral burden. *Journal of Psychosomatic Research,* 61(2), 161-168.

Snyder, B.S. (2006). The lived experience of women diagnosed with Polycystic Ovary Syndrome. *Journal of Obstetric, Gynecological & Neonatal Nursing: Clinical Scholarship for the Care of Women, Childbearing Families & Newborns,* 35(3), 385-392.

Thatcher, S.S. (2000). *PCOS: The Hidden Epidemic.* Perspectives Press, Indiana.

Wilhelm, S. (2006). *Feeling Good about the way you look: A program for Overcoming Body Image Problems.* Guilford Press: New York, NY.

Chapter 7

Baranowska, B., Radzikowska, M., Wasilewska-Dziubinska E., & Kaplinski, A. (1999) Neuropeptide, Y, leptin, galanin and insulin in women with polycystic ovary syndrome. *Gynecology and Endocrinology,* 13, 344-351.

Geraciotti TD, Liddle RA. (1988). Impaired cholecystokinin secretion in bulimia nervosa. New *England Journal of Medicine,* 319, 683-688.

Hirschberg, A.L, Nassen, S., Stridsberg, M., Bystrom, B. & Holte, J. (2004). Impaired cholecystokinin secretion and disturbed appetite regulation in women with polycystic ovary syndrome. *Gynecology and Endocrinology* 19, 79-87.

Jahanfar, S., Malelki, H., & Mosavi, A.R. (2005)Subclinical eating disorder, polycystic ovary syndrome-is there any connection between these two conditions through leptin-a twin study. *Medical Journal of Malaysia,* 60(4), 441-446.

Moran,L.J., Noakes, M.& Vlifton, P.M. (2004) Ghrelin and measures of satiety are altered in polycystic ovary syndrome but not differently affected by diet composition. *Journal of Clinical Endocrinology and Metabolism,* 893, 337-3344.

Chapter 8

American Society for Reproductive Medicine. (2006). *Medications for Inducing Ovulations: A Guide for patients.* www.asrm.org/Patients/patientbooklets/ovulation_drugs.pdf

American Society for Reproductive Medicine. (2006). *Patient's Fact Sheet: Ovulation Detection,* www.asrm.org/Patients/patientbooklets/ovulation_detection.pdf

American Society for Reproductive Medicine. (2008). *Assisted Reproductive Technologies: A Guide for Patients.* www.asrm.org/Patients/patientbooklets/ART.pdf

American Society for Reproductive Medicine. (2008.) *Patient Fact Sheet: How Doctor's Evaluate Infertility in Women.* www.asrm.org/Patients/FactSheets/InfertilityInWomen.pdf

Covington, S. & Hammer Burns, L. (2006) *Infertility Counseling: A Comprehensive Handbook for Clinicians.* Cambridge University Press: Cambridge, MA.

Grassi, A. (2007). *The Dietitian's Guide to Polycystic Ovary Syndrome.* Luca Publishing: Haverford, PA.

McCook, J.G., Reame, N.E. & Thatcher, S.S. (2006). Health-related quality of life issues in women with polycystic ovary syndrome. *Journal of Obstetric, Gynecologic, and Neonatal Nursing, 34 (1),* 12-20.

Paulus, W.E. (2002). Influence of acupuncture on the pregnancy rate in patients who undergo assisted reproduction therapy. *Fertility and Sterility, 77* (4), 721-724.

Seale, F.G., Robinson, R.D., Neal, G.S. (2000). Association of metformin and pregnancy in polycystic ovary syndrome: A report of three cases. *Journal of Reproductive Medicine, 45,* 507-510.

Sonino, N., Fava, G.A., Belluardo, P., Boscaro, M. (1993). Quality of life of hirsute women. *Postgraduate Medical Journal, 69,* 186-189.

Stener-Victorin, E., Waldenstrom, U., Tagnfors, U., Lundeberg T., & Lindstedt G., Janson P.O. (2000). Effects of electro-acupuncture on anovulation in women with polycystic ovary syndrome. *Acta Obstetricia et Gynecologica Scandinavica, 79* (3), 180-188.

Tran, N., Hunter, S., & Yankowitz, J. (2004). Oral hypoglycemic agents in pregnancy. *Obstetrical and Gynecological Survey, 59 (6),* 456-463.

Chapter 9

McCluskey, S, Lacey, J.H., Pearce, J.M. (1992). Binge-eating and polycystic ovaries. *Lancet,* 340, 723.

Michelmore, K.F., Balen, A.H. & Dunger, D.B. (2001). Polycystic ovaries and eating disorders: are they related? *Human Reproduction,* 16(4), 765-769.

Sharma, S, Nestler J (2006). Prevention of diabetes and cardiovascular disease in women with PCOS: treatment with insulin sensitizers. *Best Practice Research Clinical Endocrinology and Metabolism,* 20(2), 245-260.

APPENDIX A

PCOS LAB RESULTS TRACKING FORM

Lab Test	Optimal Levels	Date: Result	Date: Result	Date: Result	Date: Result	Date: Result	Date: Result	Date: Result	Date: Result
Total Cholesterol	< 200 mg/dL								
LDL	< 100 mg/dL								
HDL	> 55 mg/dL								
Triglycerides	< 150 mg/dL								
Fasting Glucose	70-99 mg/dL								
HA1C	< 6%								
Fasting Insulin	< 10 IU/mL								
Fasting Glucose:Insulin	> 4:5								
Total Testosterone	< 50 ng/dL								
LH	_____								
FSH	_____								
LH:FSH	1:1								
Vitamin D	> 35 ng/dL								
TSH	.4-2.5 IU/mL								
hsCRP	< 3 mg/L								
Blood Pressure	< 120/80 mmHg								

Appendix B

Food Journal

Time	Food Eaten & Amount	Grains / Starches	Protein	Fats	Fruits	Vegetables	Hunger / Satisfaction	Thoughts, feelings, symptoms
							1 2 3 4 5 6 7 8 9 10	
							1 2 3 4 5 6 7 8 9 10	
							1 2 3 4 5 6 7 8 9 10	
							1 2 3 4 5 6 7 8 9 10	
							1 2 3 4 5 6 7 8 9 10	
	Total Amount						Medication AM ☐ PM ☐	Physical Activity ☐☐☐☐☐☐☐
	Recommended Amount							

APPENDIX C

HUNGER AND SATISFACTION SCALE

1. Completely empty. Beyond starving.
2. Very hungry. You need to eat now!
3. Getting pretty hungry and will need to eat very soon.
4. Starting to feel the urge to eat.
5. Neutral. Not hungry. Not full.
6. Starting to feel like the food is enough.
7. The food is enough. Stop here and you won't be hungry again for awhile.
8. Pretty full and starting to get uncomfortable.
9. Uncomfortable. Ate too much.
10. So completely stuffed that it's painful.

APPENDIX D

RESOURCES FOR POLYCYSTIC OVARY SYNDROME

EDUCATION, ADVOCACY AND SUPPORT ORGANIZATIONS

Children's Hospital of Boston Center for Young Women's Health
www.youngwomenshealth.org/pcosinfo.html
Focuses on PCOS information for teenagers. This website has a great explanation of many common PCOS questions, featuring figures and graphs. It also includes information on reading food labels, recipes, snack ideas, sample menus and worksheets for menu planning and exercise, all specifically targeted to the PCOS teen.

PCOS Nutrition
551 W. Lancaster Avenue, #305
Haverford, PA 19041
www.PCOSnutrition.com
(484) 252-9028
The personal website for Angela Grassi, MS, RD, LDN, author of *The Dietitian's Guide to Polycystic Ovary Syndrome* and *The PCOS Workbook*. Find articles and resources on PCOS and nutrition. Angela offers nutrition counseling by phone or in person for individuals with PCOS. She also co-runs a monthly PCOS support group in the Philadelphia area. Sign up for her free newsletter, *PCOS Nutrition Tips*.

PCOS Network
www.PCOSnetwork.com
Founded by Stacey Korfist, a psychotherapist in southern California who has PCOS, this website is a wonderful resource for professionals and consumers. Use this website to find a professional in your area, articles, books and resources on PCOS. This website provides a centralized place for professionals who treat PCOS to network and collaborate.

Project PCOS
www.projectPCOS.org
Established and run by women with PCOS, this site provides awareness, information and support for women with PCOS from the top experts in the field. Find articles, recipes and information on how to be an advocate and personal stories. It is a great site to find PCOS treatment professionals and groups across the country.

PCOS Today Magazine

www.PCOStoday.net

Created and run by professor Linda Harvey who has PCOS, this online magazine is dedicated to providing up-to-date information on PCOS including causes and treatment, resources, personal stories, book reviews, question-and-answer section, and clinical trials. In addition, you can keep tabs on Linda and her perspectives on PCOS by reading her blog.

Soulcysters

www.soulcysters.net

A wonderful resource for women with PCOS. This website provides a good overview of symptoms, treatment and other PCOS links. Also provides numerous message boards depending on areas of interest where individuals can post questions and read others responses. Get book reviews and up-to-date research studies on PCOS.

Polycystic Ovary Association

www.PCOSupport.org

The Polycystic Ovary Association website includes a member database to find professionals who treat PCOS. It also has research articles and provides chat rooms for different PCOS concerns (i.e. eating disorders, infertility, etc). You can sign up for its newsletter, which includes professional interviews and book reviews.

Polycystic Ovary Syndrome of Australia

www.posaa.asn.au

This is the website for the Polycystic Ovary Syndrome of Australia. It's very similar to the Polycystic Ovary Association in the United States. This website contains support, information and advocacy for women with PCOS. The Australia website also includes chat rooms, message boards, professional database and annual conference.

Verity

www.verity-pcos.org.uk

Verity is a support organization for women with PCOS living in the United Kingdom. Use this site to find information and professionals. It has a newsletter, discussion board and fact sheets. This organization also has an annual conference.

Professional Associations

Academy for Eating Disorders

www.aedweb.org

The Academy for Eating Disorders is an international professional organization that promotes excellence in research, treatment and prevention of eating disorders. Use this site for links to professional publications on eating disorders and to locate a treatment professional.

American Dietetic Association
www.eatright.org
(800) 877-1600
The American Dietetic Association is the nation's largest organization for food and nutrition professionals. Use this site to find a registered dietitian, shop for books and gifts and search for food and nutrition information and publications.

American Association of Clinical Endocrinologists
www.aace.com
Use this site to find an endocrinologist in your area.

American College of Obstetricians and Gynecologists (ACOG)
www.acog.org
This site provides information on all aspects of women's health. Informational pamphlets on PCOS are available for purchase. This site can also be used to locate an OBGYN.

American Diabetes Association (ADA)
www.diabetes.org
A great resource for information on PCOS, insulin resistance and diabetes. This website provides a research database with current clinical trials. A nutrition section provides information, recipes, tips on eating out and making healthy food choices.

American Heart Association
www.americanheart.org
The best site for heart health. Find information fact sheets and tips on treating and preventing heart disease, diabetes, stroke and hypertension. Use this website to find recipes, articles and nutrition tips for adults and children.

American Psychological Association (APA)
www.apa.org
Use this site to find a psychologist and obtain resources and information on treating emotional problems.

American Society for Reproductive Medicine
www.asrm.org
The ASRM is a multidisciplinary organization committed to the advancement of reproductive medicine by serving as the leading advocate for patient care, research and education. ASRM has information on infertility for professionals and consumers. Use the website to find a reproductive endocrinologist in your area, information booklets and links to adoption agencies.

National Eating Disorders Association
www.edap.org
This great resource provides information and advocacy for eating disorders. Use this site to locate a treatment professional or download handouts. This organization hosts an annual conference for consumers and professionals.

RESOLVE: The National Infertility Association
www.resolve.org
RESOLVE: The National Infertility Association, established in 1974, is a non-profit organization to promote reproductive health and to ensure equal access to all family building options for men and women experiencing infertility or other reproductive disorders. Resolve provides awareness, support and information to people who are experiencing infertility.

Recommended Reading:

Mindfulness Practice

Wherever you go, there you are, by John Kabat-Zinn (1995).

The Miracle of Mindfulness, by Thich Naht Hanh (1999).

The Mindful Way through Depression, by Mark Williams, John Teasdale and Zindel Segal (2007).

Mindfulness in Plain English, by Bhante H. Gunaratana (2002).

Mindful Eating

Intuitive Eating, by Evelyn Tribole and Elyse Resch (2003).

Breaking Free from Emotional Eating, by Geneen Roth (2003).

The Appetite Awareness Workbook, by Linda Craighead (2006).

Gurze Books. Online catalog of hundreds of books specializing in eating disorders and distorted eating. www.bulilmia.com.

Alternative and Complementary Medicine Resources

The Natural Medicines Comprehensive Database
www.NaturalDatabase.com
The largest and most detailed listing of non-biased natural medicines available. This database is a great place to look up information on supplements, including specific manufacturer brands. You must pay a fee to become a member and access the database.

National Center for Complementary and Alternative Medicine
www.nccam.nih.gov
Sponsored by the National Institute of Health, this federally funded site provides information on complementary and alternative medicine. This is another great place to look up information on supplements.

APPENDIX E

SAMPLE MENUS

1400-1600 Calories

Breakfast	Example
1 Fruit	¾ cup blueberries
1-3 Grains/Starches	1 cup milk, nonfat
	1 cup plain oats, cooked
1 Fat	1 T almonds
	½ tsp cinnamon

Lunch	
1-2 Grains/Starches	½ cup chickpeas
3 Proteins	7 ½ oz. tofu
2-3 Vegetables	2 cups spinach salad with assorted vegetables
1 Fruit	orange
2 Fats	4 walnuts
	1 T sesame vinaigrette dressing

Snack	
1-2 Fats	
1 Protein	1 T peanut butter
1 Fruit	apple
	½ tsp cinnamon

Dinner	
3-5 Proteins	4 oz. skinless chicken
	1 oz. low-fat feta cheese
2 Vegetables	1 cup green beans
1-2 Fats	2 tsp canola oil
1-2 Grains/Starches	¾ cup brown rice

1400-1600 Calories, 28% Protein, 38% Carbohydrate, 34% Fat, 7% Saturated Fat, 30 grams Fiber, 2,100 mg Sodium

1600-1800 Calories

Breakfast	Example
1 Fruit	1 kiwi
1-2 Protein	2 eggs, cage-free
1-2 Grains/Starches	1 slice whole grain toast
1-2 Fats	½ T butter with plant sterols

Snack
1 Protein	1 oz. low-fat cheese
1 Bread/Starch	6 whole wheat crackers

Lunch
2-3 Vegetables	1 ½ cups romaine lettuce and assorted non-starchy vegetables
3 Proteins	3 oz. grilled chicken
1-2 Fats	1 tsp olive oil with T balsamic vinaigrette
2 Grains/Starches	1 cup low-sodium minestrone soup
	¼ cup croutons

Snack
1 Protein	⅓ cup edamame
1 Fruit	pear

Dinner
4-6 Proteins	5 oz. salmon
2 Vegetables	1 cup broccoli, steamed
1-2 Fats	1 tsp olive oil
1-2 Breads/Starches	½ cup sweet potato

Snack
1 Fat	¼ cup dark chocolate covered almonds
1 Fruit	plum

1600-1800 Calories, 27% Protein, 37% Carbohydrate, 36% Fat, 7.5% Saturated Fat, 30 grams Fiber, 2,160 mg Sodium

1800-2000 Calories

__Breakfast__	__Example__
1-2 Grains/Starches	½ cup quinoa, cooked
1 Fruit	1 small apple, chopped
1-2 Proteins	¾ cup milk, nonfat
1-2 Fats	1 T almonds
	½ tsp cinnamon

__Snack__
1 Grain/Starch	1 cup milk, nonfat, steamed
	½ tsp cinnamon
	1 T sugar-free vanilla flavoring

__Lunch__
1-2 Grains/Starches	1 whole wheat bun
3 Proteins	1 veggie burger
	1 oz. low-fat cheese
2-3 Vegetables	1 cup garden salad
1 Fruit	1 cup grapes
1-2 Fats	2 tsp olive oil with 1 T balsamic vinegar

__Snack__
1 Protein	4 oz. plain yogurt, low-fat
1 Fruit	1 peach
1 Fat	1 T flaxseed, ground

__Dinner__
2 Grains/Starches	1 cup bulgur pilaf, cooked
5 Proteins	5 oz. pork tenderloin
2-3 Vegetables	1 cup mixed vegetables, steamed
1-2 Fats	1 tsp. canola oil

1800-2000 Calories, 24% Protein, 48% Carbohydrate, 28% Fat, 6.4% Saturated Fat, 35 grams Fiber, 2,212 grams Sodium

2000-2200 Calories

Breakfast	Example
1 Fruit	1 cup raspberries
1-3 Grains/Starches	¼ cup low-sugar granola
	6 oz. plain yogurt, nonfat
1-2 Proteins	1 hard-boiled egg, cage-free

Snack

1 Protein	½ cup low-fat cottage cheese
1 Fruit	3/4 cup blueberries

Lunch

4 Proteins	1 oz. low-fat cheese
	3 oz. turkey
1-2 Grains/Starches	2 slices whole wheat bread
2-3 Vegetables	1 cup baby carrots
	2 T hummus
1 Fruit	1 ¼ cup strawberries, sliced

Snack

1-2 Fat	4 walnuts
1 Fruit	1 cup pineapple, fresh
1 Grain/Starch	2 squares dark chocolate

Dinner

4-6 Proteins	6 oz. halibut, grilled
2 Vegetables	1 cup asparagus, cooked
1-2 Fats	1 tsp olive oil
	6 almonds, slivered
1-2 Grains/Starches	1 cup wild rice, cooked

2000-2200 Calories, 25% Protein, 43% Carbohydrate, 32% Fat, 8% Saturated Fat, 41 grams Fiber, 2,190 grams Sodium

APPENDIX F

PCOS FOOD EXCHANGE LIST

Items on the left side of page, consume between 1–3 servings per meal and 1-2 servings per snack.*

GRAINS & STARCHES:
(15 grams carbohydrate each)
Whole grain, high fiber, low sugar are best.
1 slice of whole grain bread
½ whole wheat English muffin
½ whole wheat pita (6 in.)
¼ whole wheat bagel
½ whole wheat hamburger bun
1 small whole grain dinner roll
½ cup bran cereal
¾ cup unsweetened cereal
¼ cup low-sugar granola
½ cup oatmeal, plain
½ cup whole grain pasta, cooked
⅓ cup brown rice, cooked
⅓ cup whole wheat couscous, cooked
⅓ cup barley, cooked
½ cup bulgur, cooked
¼ cup spelt or kamut, cooked
3 Tbsp. wheat germ, dry
⅓ cup quinoa, cooked
½ cup corn
½ corn on the cob, large
½ cup green peas, cooked
½ cup mashed potatoes
½ baked/broiled potato, large
8-10 whole grain crackers
3 cups popcorn, plain

FRUITS (15 grams carbohydrate each)
Juice and fruit syrup should be avoided.
1 small apple, orange, peach
1 mini banana
4 apricots, fresh
1 Tbsp. raisins
¾ cup blueberries
1¼ cup strawberries
1 cup melon cubes or 1 slice
½ grapefruit, large
1 cup (about 12) grapes
2 plums
¾ cup pineapple
1 ¼ cup watermelon

MILK (12 grams carbohydrate)**
1 cup non-fat milk, any variety
6 oz. yogurt, plain or artificially sweetened

NON-STARCHY VEGGIES
(5 grams carbohydrate each)
½ cup cooked vegetables
1 cup raw vegetables

PROTEINS: (7 grams protein each)
Lean or low-fat are best. Consume several servings with all meals and snacks.*
1 oz. poultry, fish, beef, pork
1 whole egg
1 oz. cheese
½ cup (4 oz.) tofu
¼ cup ricotta/cottage cheese
1 oz. tuna
1 oz. shellfish
½ cup edamame (soybeans)

Exceptions:
1Tbsp. peanut butter = 1 protein, 2 fats
½ cup cooked beans = 1 protein, 1 starch
1 veggie burger, soy-based = 2 proteins

FATS: (5 grams fat each)
Avoid trans fats and limit saturated fats.*
1 tsp. oil
1 tsp. margarine/butter
1 tsp. regular mayo
1 Tbsp. cream cheese
1 slice bacon
2 Tbsp. half & half or cream
2 Tbsp. sour cream
1 Tbsp. salad dressing
1 Tbsp. sesame seeds
2 Tbsp. avocado
8 olives
10 peanuts
4 walnut halves
6 whole almonds
6 cashews
16 pistachios
2 tsp. peanut/almond butter
1 Tbsp. flax seed, ground

*These are approximate amounts. To find amounts for your specific needs consult with a registered dietitian.
**Although milk is a great protein source, it is also a source of carbohydrates.

ABOUT THE AUTHORS

Angela Grassi, MS, RD, LDN

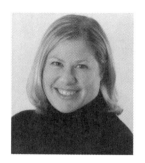

Angela Grassi, MS, RD, LDN is the author of *The Dietitian's Guide to Polycystic Ovary Syndrome*. As a registered and licensed dietitian, she provides nutrition counseling by phone or in-person to women with PCOS and individuals who struggle with Eating Disorders. In 2000, she won the award for excellence in graduate research from The American Dietetic Association. Having PCOS herself, Angela has been dedicated to the advocacy, education, and research of the syndrome. She provides lectures to dietitians, other health care professionals and women with PCOS across the country. Angela resides in the Philadelphia suburbs with her husband and son. For more information about nutrition for PCOS or to sign up for her free *PCOS Nutrition Tips newsletter*, visit www.PCOSnutrition.com.

Stephanie Mattei, Psy.D.

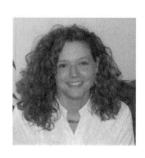

Stephanie Mattei, Psy.D. is a licensed clinical psychologist who co-founded the Center for Acceptance and Change in Bala Cynwyd, PA. She has been intensively trained in Dialectical Behavior Therapy (DBT) and teaches as adjunct faculty in the doctoral program at La Salle University in Philadelphia. She has a particular interest in working with women who struggle with Eating Disorders, PCOS, Borderline Personality Disorder, self-harm behaviors and relationship distress. Stephanie has written chapters in *The Dietitian's Guide to PCOS* and *Psychotherapists Revealed: Therapists Speak About Self-Disclosure in Psychotherapy*. Stephanie lives in the suburbs of Philadelphia with her husband and two daughters. For more information about her practice, visit www.centerforaccetpanceandchange.com.

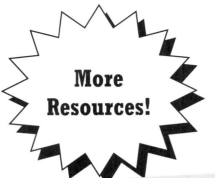
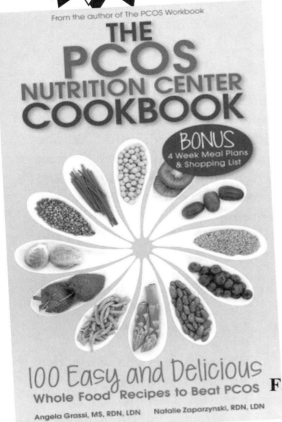
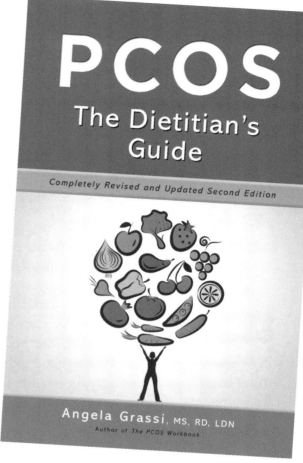
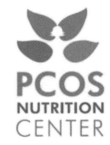